# Hypoglycemia in Diabetes

Pathophysiology, Prevalence, and Prevention

Philip E. Cryer, MD

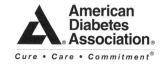
American
Diabetes
Association®
Cure • Care • Commitment®

*Director, Book Publishing,* Robert Anthony; *Managing Editor, Book Publishing,* Abe Ogden; *Acquisitions Editor, Professional Books,* Victor Van Beuren; *Editor,* Wendy Martin; *Production Manager,* Melissa Sprott; *Composition,* ADA; *Cover Design,* Koncept , Inc.; *Printer,* Thomson-Shore, Inc.

Printed in the United States of America
1 3 5 7 9 10 8 6 4 2

The suggestions and information contained in this publication are generally consistent with the *Clinical Practice Recommendations* and other policies of the American Diabetes Association, but they do not represent the policy or position of the Association or any of its boards or committees. Reasonable steps have been taken to ensure the accuracy of the information presented. However, the American Diabetes Association cannot ensure the safety or efficacy of any product or service described in this publication. Individuals are advised to consult a physician or other appropriate health care professional before undertaking any diet or exercise program or taking any medication referred to in this publication. Professionals must use and apply their own professional judgment, experience, and training and should not rely solely on the information contained in this publication before prescribing any diet, exercise, or medication. The American Diabetes Association—its officers, directors, employees, volunteers, and members—assumes no responsibility or liability for personal or other injury, loss, or damage that may result from the suggestions or information in this publication.

⊗ The paper in this publication meets the requirements of the ANSI Standard Z39.48-1992 (permanence of paper).

ADA titles may be purchased for business or promotional use or for special sales. To purchase more than 50 copies of this book at a discount, or for custom editions of this book with your logo, contact the American Diabetes Association at the address below, at booksales@diabetes.org, or by calling 703-299-2046.

American Diabetes Association
1701 North Beauregard Street
Alexandria, Virginia 22311

**Library of Congress Cataloging-in-Publication Data**

Cryer, Philip E., 1940-
  Hypoglycemia in diabetes : pathophysiology, prevalence, and prevention / Philip E. Cryer.
    p. ; cm.
  Includes bibliographical references and index.
  ISBN 978-1-58040-326-9 (alk. paper)
  1. Hypoglycemia. 2. Diabetes--Treatment--Complications. I. American Diabetes Association. II. Title.
  [DNLM: 1. Hypoglycemia--physiopathology. 2. Diabetes Complications. 3. Hypoglycemia--etiology. 4. Hypoglycemia--prevention & control. WK 880 C957h 2009]
  RC662.2.C79 2009
  616.4'66--dc22

                        2008049690

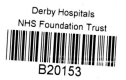

*This book is dedicated to the research nurses, led for a quarter of a century by Carolyn E. Havlin-Cryer, RN, and the following research fellows:*

Alan J. Garber, MD, PhD
William L. Clarke, MD
Alan B. Silverberg, MD
Steven A. Leveston, MD
Jack F. Tohmeh, MD
William E. Clutter, MD
Dennis A. Popp, MD
Ann M. Ginsberg, MD, PhD
Pierre Serusclat, MD
Thomas F. Tse, MD
Stephen G. Rosen, MD
Michael A. Berk, MD
Myrlene Staten, MD
David P. Hoelzer, MD
Natalie S. Schwartz, MD
Katherine R. Tuttle, MD
Karen M. Tordjman, MD
Stephen B. Liggett, MD
James C. Marker, PhD
Patrick J. Boyle, MD

Irl B. Hirsch, MD
Simon R. Heller, DM, FRCP
Brian V. Wiethop, MD
Samuel E. Dagogo-Jack, MB/BS
Dwight A. Towler, MD, PhD
Chatchalit Rattarasarn, MD
Annemarie Hvidberg, MD, PhD
Tarek Saleh, MD
Carmine G. Fanelli, MD
Deanna Paramore, MD
Fernando Ovalle, MD
Scott A. Segel, MD
Salomon Banarer, MD
Veronica P. McGregor, MD
Michael A. DeRosa, DO
Bharathi Raju, MD
Denise Teves, MD
Ana Maria Arbelaez, MD
Suzanne M. Breckenridge, MD
Benjamin A. Cooperberg, MD

*These individuals did the bulk of our work.*

# CONTENTS

# PREFACE

D iabetes mellitus is an increasingly common disease (Wild et al. 2004; Amos et al. 1997). It has been estimated that the prevalence of diabetes will rise from 171 million people in the year 2000 to 336 million people worldwide by the year 2030 (Wild et al. 2004). The common forms of the disease are type 1 diabetes mellitus, the result of absolute insulin deficiency from its clinical onset, and type 2 diabetes mellitus, the result of relative insulin deficiency in the setting of insulin resistance early in its course and absolute insulin deficiency later. More than 95% of affected people have type 2 diabetes (Amos et al. 1997).

Over time, diabetes can cause unique microvascular complications—retinopathy, nephropathy, and neuropathy—and a substantially increased risk for macrovascular atherosclerotic complications—myocardial infarction, cerebrovascular accidents, and peripheral vascular disease. These long-term complications are undoubtedly multifactorial in origin, but it is now well established, at least for microvascular disease, that hyperglycemia is one important factor (Diabetes Control and Complications Trial Research Group [DCCT] 1993; Diabetes Control and Complications Trial/Epidemiology of Diabetes Interventions and Complications Research Group 2000, 2005; U.K. Prospective Diabetes Study Group [UKPDS] 1998a, 1998b; Holman et al. 2008). Therefore, maintenance of plasma glucose concentrations closer to the nondiabetic range prevents or delays these complications. Indeed, it is conceivable that maintenance of normal plasma glucose concentrations over a lifetime of diabetes would eliminate the microvascular complications (DCCT 1995) and reduce the risk of macrovascular disease substantially (Stettler et al. 2006).

Unfortunately, with current treatment regimens, it is not possible to maintain euglycemia over a lifetime of diabetes in the vast majority of people with diabetes because of the barrier of iatrogenic (treatment-induced) hypoglycemia (Cryer 1997, 2001, 2004, 2008). Pending the prevention and cure of diabetes, maintenance of euglycemia without hypoglycemia will require new treatment methods that provide plasma glucose–regulated insulin replacement or secretion.

The biochemistry, physiology, and pathophysiology of intermediary metabolism, with a focus on glucoregulation and hypoglycemia, have been reviewed (Cryer 1997, 2001, 2004, 2008), and the history of hypoglycemia in the 20th century has been summarized (Cryer 1997). The impact of hypoglycemia was first documented in 1921 when a dog convulsed and then died after injection of extracted insulin; hypoglycemia was recognized to be a complication of insulin treatment of diabetes shortly thereafter (Bliss 1992).

In this book, the term "hypoglycemia" is used to refer to both clinical and physiological hypoglycemia. Those are different. Unequivocal demonstration of clinical hypoglycemia requires documentation of Whipple's triad (Whipple 1938): symptoms, signs, or both consistent with hypoglycemia, a reliably measured low–plasma glucose concentration, and resolution of those symptoms and signs after the plasma glucose level is raised (Cryer 1997, 2001, 2004; Cryer et al. In press). In healthy individuals, symptoms of hypoglycemia develop at an arterialized venous plasma glucose concentration of ~54 mg/dl (~3.0 mmol/l) (Cryer 2001). From a physiological perspective, however, the glycemic threshold is at a higher glucose level. Arterialized venous plasma glucose concentrations just below the postabsorptive physiological range, i.e., <70 mg/dl (<3.9 mmol/l), trigger physiological defenses against falling plasma glucose concentrations including further decrements in the secretion of insulin and initial increments in the secretion of glucose counterregulatory hormones such as glucagon and epinephrine (Cryer 2001). Indeed, the latter higher plasma glucose concentration, with or without symptoms, has been recommended as a pragmatic alert level for people with diabetes who are at high risk for clinical hypoglycemia (American Diabetes Association Workgroup on Hypoglycemia 2005).

The clinical problem of iatrogenic hypoglycemia in diabetes is the subject of this book. The problem is approached from the perspective of the pathophysiology of glucose counterregulation, the mechanisms that normally effectively prevent or correct hypoglycemia (Cryer 2001), in type 1 diabetes and advanced type 2 diabetes (Cryer 1997, 2004, 2008). The premise is that insight into that pathophysiology leads to understanding of the frequency of, risk factors for, and prevention of iatrogenic hypoglycemia in people with diabetes.

# ACKNOWLEDGMENTS

The author's original work cited has been supported in part by the U.S. Public Health Service, National Institutes of Health grants, including R37 DK27085, MO1 RR00036, P60 DK20579, and T32 DK07120, and by a fellowship award from the American Diabetes Association. The author is grateful for the contributions of his mentors, collaborators, and colleagues; the efforts of the postdoctoral fellows who did the bulk of the work and made the work better by their conceptual input; and the skilled nursing, technical, dietary, and data management/statistical assistance of the staff of the Washington University General Clinical Research Center. Ms. Janet Dedeke prepared this manuscript.

Thanks to M. Sue Kirkman, MD, and Stephen N. Davis, MD, for their review of this manuscript.

## DISCLOSURES

The author has served as a consultant to several pharmaceutical or medical device firms, including Amgen Inc., Johnson & Johnson, MannKind Corp., Marcadia Biotech, Medtronic MiniMed Inc., Merck and Co., Novo Nordisk A/S, Takeda Pharmaceuticals North America, and TolerRx Inc.

# Chapter 1.
# The Clinical Problem of Hypoglycemia in Diabetes

Iatrogenic hypoglycemia is the limiting factor in the glycemic management of diabetes (Cryer 2004, 2008). First, it causes recurrent morbidity in most people with type 1 diabetes, and many with advanced type 2 diabetes, and is sometimes fatal. Second, it compromises physiological and behavioral defenses against subsequent falling plasma glucose concentrations and thus causes a vicious cycle of recurrent hypoglycemia. Third, it precludes maintenance of euglycemia over a lifetime of diabetes and thus full realization of the microvascular and potential macrovascular benefits of long-term glycemic control (DCCT 1993; Diabetes Control and Complications Trial/Epidemiology of Diabetes Interventions and Complications Group 2000, 2005; UKPDS 1998a, 1998b; Holman et al. 2008). Because of the barrier of hypoglycemia, no professional treatment guidelines recommend a glycemic goal of euglycemia, i.e., a normal hemoglobin A1c (A1C) level, although that would undoubtedly be beneficial with respect to the long-term complications of diabetes (DCCT 1993; Diabetes Control and Complications Trial/Epidemiology of Diabetes Interventions and Complications Group 2000, 2005; UKPDS 1998a, 1998b; Holman et al. 2008) if it could be accomplished safely. For example, the American Diabetes Association (American Diabetes Association

**1**

[ADA] 2008) recommends an A1C goal of <7% for patients in general and "as close to normal (<6%) as possible without significant hypoglycemia" for selected individual patients.

Glucose is an obligate metabolic fuel for the brain under physiological conditions (Cryer 2001, 2004, 2007, 2008). Mechanisms have evolved that normally very effectively prevent or rapidly correct hypoglycemia despite wide variations in glucose flux into and out of the circulation (Cryer 2001, 2004, 2007, 2008) (Chapter 2) undoubtedly because of their survival value. Thus, hypoglycemia is a distinctly uncommon clinical event, except in people who use drugs that lower the plasma glucose concentration, particularly insulin or an insulin secretagogue, to treat diabetes (Cryer 2004).

Clinical hypoglycemia is a plasma glucose concentration low enough to cause symptoms and/or signs, including impairment of brain function. Because the clinical manifestations of hypoglycemia are nonspecific (Chapter 2), hypoglycemia is documented most convincingly by Whipple's triad (Whipple 1938): symptoms, signs, or both consistent with hypoglycemia, a low plasma glucose concentration, and resolution of the symptoms and signs after the plasma glucose concentration is raised (Cryer 2008; Cryer et al. In press).

Hypoglycemia in diabetes is generally the result of the interplay of relative or absolute therapeutic (exogenous or endogenous) insulin excess and compromised physiological and behavioral defenses against falling plasma glucose concentrations (Cryer 2004, 2008) (Chapter 3). Thus, it is fundamentally iatrogenic, the result of treatments that raise circulating insulin levels and therefore lower plasma glucose concentrations. Those treatments include insulin or an insulin secretagogue such as a sulfonylurea (glyburide [glibenclamide], glipizide, or glimepiride, among others) or a non-sulfonylurea (nateglinide or repaglinide). All people with type 1 diabetes must be treated with insulin. Most people with type 2 diabetes ultimately require treatment with insulin. Early in the course of type 2 diabetes, patients may respond to an insulin secretagogue, with the risk of hypoglycemia. Alternatively, they may respond to drugs that do not raise insulin levels at normal or low plasma glucose concentrations and therefore should not, and probably do not (Bolen et al. 2007), cause hypoglycemia. The latter include the biguanide metformin—which nonetheless has been reported to cause self-reported hypoglycemia (UKPDS 1995; Wright et al. 2006)—thiazolidinediones (e.g., pioglitazone, rosiglitazone), $\alpha$-glucosidase inhibitors (e.g., acarbose, miglitol), glucagon-like peptide-1 (GLP-1) receptor agonists (e.g., exenatide, liraglutide), and dipeptidyl peptidase-IV (DPP-IV) inhibitors (e.g., sitagliptin, vildagliptin). All of these drugs require endogenous insulin secretion to lower plasma glucose concentrations, and insulin secretion declines appropriately as glucose levels fall into the normal range. That is true even for the GLP-1 receptor agonists and the DPP-IV inhibitors, which enhance glucose-stimulated insulin secretion (among other actions). They do not stimulate insulin secretion at normal or low plasma glucose levels (i.e., they increase insulin secretion in a glucose-dependent fashion). However, the latter feature may be lost, and hypoglycemia can occur, when GLP-1 receptor agonists and DPP-IV inhibitors are used with an insulin secretagogue (de Heer and Holst 2007). Indeed, all five categories of drugs—biguanides, thiazolidinediones, $\alpha$-glucosidase inhibitors, GLP-1 receptor agonists, and DPP-IV inhibitors—increase the risk of hypoglycemia if used with an insulin secretagogue or with insulin.

**Table 1.1** Event Rates for Severe Hypoglycemia (that Requiring the Assistance of Another Person), Expressed as Episodes per 100 Patient-Years, in Insulin-Treated Diabetes

| | n | Event rate | Comment |
|---|---|---|---|
| **Type 1 Diabetes** | | | |
| U.K. Hypoglycaemia Study Group 2007 | 57[a] 50[b] | 320 110 | Prospective multicenter study |
| MacLeod et al. 1993 | 544 | 170 | Retrospective clinic survey, randomly selected sample |
| Donnelly et al. 2005 | 94 | 115 | Prospective study, population-based random sample |
| Reichard and Pihl 1994 | 48 | 110 | Clinical trial, intensive insulin group |
| DCCT Research Group 1993 | 711 | 62 | Clinical trial, intensive insulin group |
| **Type 2 Diabetes** | | | |
| MacLeod et al. 1993 | 56 | 73 | Retrospective clinic survey, randomly selected sample |
| U.K. Hypoglycaemia Study Group 2007 | 77[c] 89[d] | 70 10 | Prospective multicenter study |
| Akram et al. 2006 | 401 | 44 | Retrospective clinic survey |
| Donnelly et al. 2005 | 173 | 35 | Prospective study, population-based random sample |
| Henderson et al. 2003 | 215 | 28 | Retrospective clinic survey, randomly selected sample |
| Murata et al. 2005 | 344 | 21 | Prospective study, random Veterans Affairs sample |
| Saudek et al. 1996 | 62 | 18[e] | Clinical trial, multiple insulin injection group |
| Gürlek et al. 1999 | 114 | 15 | Retrospective clinic survey |
| Abraira et al. 1995 | 75 | 3 | Clinical trial, intensive insulin group |
| Yki-Järvinen et al. 1999 | 88 | 0 | Clinical trial, initial insulin therapy |
| Ohkubo et al. 1995 | 52 | 0 | Clinical trial, initial insulin therapy |

[a]Insulin treatment for >15 years
[b]Insulin treatment for <5 years
[c]Insulin treatment for >5 years
[d]Insulin treatment for <2 years
[e]Definite (8 per 100 patient-years) plus suspected (10 per 100 patient-years) severe hypoglycemia

Studies covering at least 1 year, involving at least 48 patients, and reporting severe hypoglycemia event rates are included. This table was prepared, by the author, for a Clinical Practice Guideline on hypoglycemia in adults (Cryer et al. In press).

Because of the difficulty of ascertainment, reported incidences of hypoglycemia in diabetes are generally underestimates. Asymptomatic episodes of hypoglycemia will be missed unless they are detected by routine self–plasma glucose monitoring (or by reliable continuous glucose sensing). Because the symptoms of hypoglycemia are nonspecific (Chapter 2), symptomatic episodes may not be recognized as the result of hypoglycemia (Clarke et al. 1995). Even if they are recognized, mild-to-moderate self-treated episodes are often not long remembered (Pramming et al. 1991; Pedersen-Bjergaard et al. 2003) and therefore may not be reported accurately at periodic clinic visits. Episodes of severe hypoglycemia (those so sufficiently disabling that they require the assistance of another person) are more dramatic events that are much more likely to be recalled (Pramming et al. 1991; Pedersen-Bjergaard et al. 2003) and therefore reported (by the patient or by a close associate). Thus, although they represent only a small fraction of the total hypoglycemic experience, estimates of the incidence of severe hypoglycemia are the most reliable. (Arguably, they are also most important, since they pose a high risk for a subsequent serious adverse outcome and dictate consideration of a major change in the therapeutic regimen.) In addition, hypoglycemia event rates determined prospectively, particularly if hypoglycemia is the primary outcome in a population-based study, should be more reliable than those determined retrospectively.

While estimates of the incidence of hypoglycemia (Table 1.1) are often derived from clinical treatment trials, there are several limitations to that approach. First, hypoglycemia is not a primary outcome of such trials; therefore, the extent of collection of data concerning hypoglycemia varies. For example, much was learned about the incidence of hypoglycemia in type 1 diabetes in the

DCCT (DCCT 1997), but the incidence of hypoglycemia in type 2 diabetes in the U.K. Prospective Diabetes Study (UKPDS) is not known (Wright et al. 2006). Second, treatment trials in type 2 diabetes are often conducted in patients just failing oral hypoglycemic agent therapy and naive to insulin therapy. Such patients are not representative of advanced type 2 diabetes and are at relatively low risk for hypoglycemia, as mentioned earlier (UK Hypo Group 2007), for pathophysiological reasons developed in Chapter 3. Third, if used exclusively, that approach ignores evidence from clinical experience in diabetes specialist clinics and, particularly, data from prospective, population-based studies focused on hypoglycemia.

The prospective, population-based study of Donnelly and colleagues (Donnelly et al. 2005) indicates that the overall incidence of hypoglycemia in insulin-treated type 2 diabetes is approximately one-third of that in type 1 diabetes (Table 1.1). In patients with type 1 diabetes, the event rates for any hypoglycemia and for severe hypoglycemia were ~4,300 per 100 patient years and 115 per 100 patient-years, respectively. In patients with insulin-treated type 2 diabetes, the event rates for any hypoglycemia and for severe hypoglycemia were ~1,600 per 100 patient years and 35 per 100 patient-years, respectively. Furthermore, in population-based studies from single hospital regions with known incidences of type 1 diabetes and type 2 diabetes, event rates for severe hypoglycemia requiring emergency medical treatment in insulin-treated type 2 diabetes were ~40% (Holstein et al. 2003) and ~100% (Leese et al. 2003) of those in type 1 diabetes. Because the prevalence of type 2 diabetes is ~20-fold greater than that of type 1 diabetes (Amos et al. 1997), and because most people with type 2 diabetes ultimately require treatment with insulin, these data suggest that most episodes of iatrogenic hypoglycemia, including severe iatrogenic hypoglycemia, occur in people with type 2 diabetes. Clearly, the magnitude of the problem of hypoglycemia in type 2 diabetes should not be underestimated.

In summary, compared with that in type 1 diabetes, the incidence of hypoglycemia is relatively low (at least with currently recommended glycemic goals) during treatment with an insulin secretagogue or even with insulin early in the course of type 2 diabetes (UK Hypo Group 2007). However, hypoglycemia becomes progressively more frequent, with its incidence approaching that in type 1 diabetes, in longstanding insulin-treated type 2 diabetes (UK Hypo Group 2007). As developed in Chapter 3, this increase in the frequency of iatrogenic hypoglycemia parallels progressive β-cell failure in type 2 diabetes and thus development of the pathophysiology of glucose counterregulation—compromised physiological and behavioral defenses against falling plasma glucose concentrations—as patients approach the insulin-deficient end of the spectrum of type 2 diabetes (Cryer 2004, 2008).

## IMPACT OF HYPOGLYCEMIA

Iatrogenic hypoglycemia causes recurrent morbidity in most people with type 1 diabetes and many with advanced type 2 diabetes and is sometimes fatal (Cryer 2004, 2008). Because it precludes maintenance of euglycemia over a lifetime of diabetes, and thus full realization not only of the microvascular benefits (DCCT 1993, 2000; UKPDS 1998a, 1998b), but also of the apparent long-term macrovascular benefits (Diabetes Control and Complications Trial/Epidemiology of Diabetes Interventions and Complications Group 2005; Holman et al. 2008) of glycemic control, the barrier of hypoglycemia may also contribute to the most prevalent cause of disabling morbidity and of mortality in diabetes—cardiovascular disease.

## Morbidity

Glucose, derived almost exclusively from the circulation, is an obligate metabolic fuel for the brain under physiological conditions (Chapter 2). Hypoglycemia causes brain fuel deprivation that, if unchecked, results in functional brain failure that is typically corrected after the plasma glucose concentration is raised (Cryer 2007). Rarely, profound, prolonged hypoglycemia results in brain death (Cryer 2007).

The physical morbidity of an episode of hypoglycemia ranges from unpleasant symptoms, such as palpitations, tremulousness, anxiety, sweating, hunger, and paresthesias (Towler et al. 1993), and cognitive impairments with behavioral changes to seizure, coma, or, rarely, death (Cryer 2007). Physical injuries or transient focal neurological deficits occur rarely. Seemingly complete recovery after an episode of hypoglycemia is the rule. Permanent neurological damage is rare. In monkeys, 5–6 hours of blood glucose concentrations <20 mg/dl (1.1 mmol/l) were required for the regular production of brain damage (Kahn and Myers 1971).

While there is ongoing concern that recurrent hypoglycemic episodes might cause permanent cognitive impairments, particularly in young children (Hershey et al. 2005), the results of long-term follow-up of DCCT patients (Diabetes Control and Complications Trial/Epidemiology of Diabetes Interventions and Complications Study Research Group 2007) are to a large extent reassuring. In 1,144 patients with type 1 diabetes (40% of whom suffered at least one episode of hypoglycemic coma or seizure) followed for a mean of 18 years, hypoglycemia was not associated with a decline in any cognitive domain (Diabetes Control and Complications Trial/Epidemiology of Diabetes Interventions and Complications Study Research Group 2007). Nonetheless, in children with type 1 diabetes, repeated severe hypoglycemia, particularly that beginning before the age of 5 years, has been associated with impaired spatial long-term memory performance (Hershey et al. 2005). It is also associated with smaller left superior temporal gray matter volume, as measured with magnetic resonance imaging (Perantie et al. 2007). Thus, with the patient who dies from hypoglycemia aside, recurrent hypoglycemia does not appear to cause cognitive impairment in young to middle-aged adults with type 1 diabetes (Diabetes Control and Complications Trial/Epidemiology of Diabetes Interventions and Complications Study Research Group 2007). Evidence that it does not do so in elderly patients is lacking (both the Action to Control Cardiovascular Risk in Diabetes [ACCORD] trial and the Veterans Affairs Diabetes Trial [VADT] have cognitive testing as part of their protocols, so this will be coming), and the distinct possibility that it does so in children remains (Hershey et al. 2005; Perantie et al. 2007).

At the very least, an episode of hypoglycemia is a nuisance and a distraction. Hypoglycemia can be embarrassing and lead to social ostracism or employment discrimination. It can be mistaken for alcohol intoxication or illicit drug use. The resulting aberrant behavior and impaired judgment can lead to offensive acts, and altered psychomotor functions can cause impaired performance of physical tasks (such as driving). The psychological morbidity of iatrogenic hypoglycemia includes fear of an episode (which can be a major barrier to glycemic control), guilt about that fear, higher levels of anxiety, and lower levels of overall happiness (Jacobsen 1996).

## Mortality

Profound, prolonged hypoglycemia can cause brain death, but in other instances, the mechanism of death is unclear (Cryer 2007). Cardiac arrhythmias are a possible mechanism (Lee et al. 2004; Laitenen et al. 2008; Adler et al. In press). Hypoglycemia causes a transiently prolonged corrected QT interval (QTc), among other electrocardiographic changes (Lee et al. 2004; Laitenen et al. 2008). These changes are thought to be mediated by the increased sympathoadrenal activity triggered by hypoglycemia. Furthermore, recent antecedent hypoglycemia causes subsequent reduced baroreflex sensitivity (Adler et al. In press). These alterations have been associated with ventricular arrhythmias, a plausible mechanism of hypoglycemia-induced sudden death. Regardless of the precise mechanism, there is a hypoglycemic mortality rate in type 1 diabetes and type 2 diabetes. Earlier studies reported that 2–4% of patients with insulin-treated diabetes (mostly type 1 diabetes) died from hypoglycemia (Deckert et al. 1978; Tunbridge 1981). More recent studies report similar hypoglycemia mortality rates (Laing et al. 1999; Skrivarhaug et al. 2006; Feltbower et al. 2008). For example, 10% (10 of 103) (Skrivarhaug et al. 2006) and 7% (8 of 108) (Feltbower et al. 2008) of deaths of patients with type 1 diabetes were attributed to hypoglycemia. Three of the 53 deaths in the DCCT cohort of 1,144 patients with type 1 diabetes followed for a mean of 18 years were attributed to hypoglycemia (Diabetes Control and Complications Trial/Epidemiology of Diabetes Interventions and Complications Study Research Group 2007.). Among people with type 2 diabetes and severe sulfonylurea-induced hypoglycemia, death rates ranging up to 10% have been reported (Gerich 1989; Holstein and Egberts 2003).

Hyperglycemia is common in critically ill patients, even individuals without diabetes. As expected, aggressive glycemic therapy has been found to result in an increased frequency of hypoglycemia in randomized controlled trials in such patients (Van den Berghe et al. 2001, 2006; Brunkhorst et al. 2008). While death during hypoglycemia was not observed in the published trials, hypoglycemia was identified as a risk factor for death (Van den Berghe et al. 2006; Brunkhorst et al. 2008). Many of the initially reported morbidity benefits and the mortality benefit of maintenance of plasma glucose concentrations in the 80–110 mg/dl (4.4–6.1 mmol/l) range in critically ill patients (Van den Berghe et al. 2001) have not been confirmed in other randomized controlled trials (Van den Berghe et al. 2006; Brunkhorst et al. 2008). Thus, whereas some degree of glycemic control is reasonable, the goal of euglycemia seems difficult to justify on the basis of the risk-to-benefit relationship (Cryer 2006; Preiser and Devos 2007).

The ACCORD randomized controlled trial provided further evidence that there is a limit to the degree of glycemic control that can be accomplished safely with currently available treatment methods (Action to Control Cardiovascular Risk in Diabetes Study Group [ACCORD] 2008). In the ACCORD trial, patients with type 2 diabetes at high cardiovascular risk were randomized to intensive glycemic therapy ($n$ = 5,128) or standard glycemic therapy ($n$ = 5,123); stable median A1C values were 6.4 and 7.5%, respectively. After a median of 3.4 years, 257 (5.0%) patients in the intensive therapy group and 203 (4.0%) patients in the standard therapy group had died, and intensive therapy was discontinued. The cause, or causes, of excess mortality during more intensive therapy is not known (ACCORD 2008). It could have been chance; excess mortality was not observed in another large trial of intensive glycemic therapy in type 2 diabetes with a similar median A1C (6.4%), albeit with less glycemic separation between the groups (median A1C of 7.0% in the standard therapy group) (ADVANCE Collaborative Group [ADVANCE] 2008). It could have been the result of nonglycemic effects of the intensive regimen (drugs, weight gain, other). However, the most plausible cause of excess mortality in the ACCORD trial is hypoglycemia: *1*) Mean glycemia (A1C) was intentionally and demonstrably lower. *2*) Lower mean glycemia (A1C) is associated with a higher prevalence of hypoglycemia (Wright et al. 2006; ACCORD 2008; ADVANCE 2008). *3*) Hypoglycemia can be fatal (including sudden, presumably cardiac arrhythmic, death as well as brain death) (Cryer 2007; Lee et al. 2004; Adler et al. In press). *4*) More patients died in the group with lower mean glycemia (ACCORD 2008). The absence of direct evidence (plasma glucose measurements just before the 460 deaths in the ACCORD trial) precludes an unequivocal conclusion that hypoglycemia was or was not a culprit. But the absence of indirect evidence of an association between hypoglycemia and excess mortality cannot justify a categorical conclusion that hypoglycemia was not a culprit.

## SUMMARY

Hypoglycemia is a problem for many people with diabetes that has not been solved. It is fundamentally iatrogenic, the result of therapeutic hyperinsulinemia. However, because of the effectiveness of normal defenses against falling plasma glucose concentrations (Chapter 2), hypoglycemia is relatively uncommon early in the course of type 2 diabetes (and is uncommon very early—the "honeymoon" period—in type 1 diabetes). However, hypoglycemia becomes more common over time as those defenses become compromised (Chapter 3). Understanding the latter pathophysiology leads to insight into the risk factors for (Chapter 4), definition and classification of (Chapter 5), and prevention or treatment of (Chapter 6) iatrogenic hypoglycemia in diabetes.

# Chapter 2.
# The Physiology of
# Glucose Counterregulation

Glucose is an obligate oxidative fuel for the brain under physiological conditions (Clarke and Sokoloff 1994; Cryer 2007, 2008). Although the adult human brain constitutes only ~2% of body weight, it accounts for >50% of whole-body glucose utilization. Thus, survival of the brain, and therefore the individual, requires a virtually continuous supply of glucose to the brain.

Neurons normally oxidize lactate as well as glucose, but that is lactate derived from glucose within the brain—mostly glucose transported from the circulation into the brain but partly that derived from glycogen in astrocytes (Itoh et al. 2003; Hyder et al. 2006). The brain can use fuels other than glucose from the circulation if their circulating levels rise high enough to enter the brain in quantity (a commonly cited example is ketone bodies that are elevated during prolonged fasting [Owen et al. 1969]), but that is seldom the case. The fact remains that among the potential substrates that normally circulate, including lactate and β-hydroxybutyrate, only injection of glucose has been found to rescue the brain of a hypoglycemic animal (Clarke and Sokoloff 1994).

At elevated, physiological, or even slightly subphysiological (e.g., 65 mg/dl [3.6 mmol/l]) plasma glucose concentrations, the rate of blood-to-brain glucose transport exceeds the rate of brain glucose metabolism (Fanelli et al. 1998; Segel et al. 2001). Thus, all of the glucose required to provide oxidative fuel to the brain can be accounted for by glucose from the circulation (Wahren et al. 1999; Lubow et al. 2006). The balance of the glucose transported into the brain is either stored as (astrocytic) glycogen or transported back into the circulation.

Direct studies of human brain substrate utilization during hypoglycemia are limited. In a study of rather brief (<40 minutes) but substantial (43 mg/dl [2.4 mmol/l]) hypoglycemia in healthy humans, brain glucose uptake accounted for ~90% of brain oxygen consumption, and there was no net uptake of lactate or pyruvate, β-hydroxybutyrate, or any of nine amino acids (Wahren et al. 1999). In another study of more sustained (<120 minutes) and nearly as substantial (54 mg/dl [3.0 mmol/l]) hypoglycemia in healthy humans, brain lactate uptake increased slightly, but that accounted for no more than 25% of the calculated brain energy deficit (Lubow et al. 2006). There was no net uptake of alanine or leucine (Lubow et al. 2006).

At some level of hypoglycemia—perhaps ~54 mg/dl (~3.0 mmol/l), since symptoms develop in healthy humans at about that level (Schwartz et al. 1987; Mitrakou et al. 1991; Fanelli et al. 1994a)—when the rate of blood-to-brain glucose transport becomes limiting to that of brain glucose metabolism, astrocytic glycogen could be a reserve source of glucose that fuels astrocytes and (largely as lactate produced by glycolysis of glycogen-derived glucose) neurons (Öz et al. 2007). However, that reserve is limited. The brain glycogen concentration is ~1% of that in liver and 10% of that in skeletal muscle. Based on rates of brain glucose metabolism measured with [1-¹¹C] glucose and positron emission tomography in healthy humans of 0.17 μmol · g⁻¹ · min⁻¹ (Fanelli et al. 1998; Segel et al. 2001) and a brain glycogen content measured with [1-¹³C]glucose and nuclear magnetic resonance spectroscopy in healthy humans of 3.5 μmol/g glucosyl units (Öz et al. 2007), one can calculate that glycogen in the adult human brain could support brain oxidative metabolism for ~20 minutes if brain glycogen were to become the sole source of glucose (and thus lactate). Even if blood-to-brain glucose transport were to account for 90% of brain glucose metabolism during mild-to-moderate hypoglycemia (Fanelli et al. 1998; Segel et al. 2001; Wahren et al. 1999; Lubow et al. 2006), the 10% supply of brain glycogen-derived glucose (and lactate) would be exhausted in ~200 minutes.

In summary, because it cannot synthesize glucose, use physiological levels of circulating non-glucose fuels effectively, or store more than 20 minutes' supply as glycogen, the brain requires a virtually continuous supply of glucose from the circulation. Because facilitated blood-to-brain glucose transport (mediated by glucose transporter-1) is a direct function of the arterial plasma glucose concentration, maintenance of the plasma glucose concentration at or above the normal range is required. At low plasma glucose concentrations, functional brain failure (and, if hypoglycemia is profound and prolonged, brain death) occurs (Cryer 2007).

## RESPONSES TO HYPOGLYCEMIA

Falling plasma glucose concentrations elicit a characteristic sequence of responses in humans (Schwartz et al. 1987; Mitra-

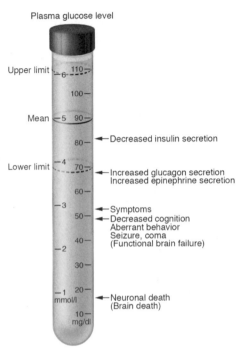

**Figure 2.1.** Sequence of responses to falling plasma glucose concentrations in humans. From Cryer 2007, with permission from the American Society for Clinical Investigation.

kou et al. 1991; Fanelli et al. 1994a). These are shown diagrammatically in Figure 2.1 and are detailed in Table 2.1. The earliest physiological response is a decrease in insulin secretion. That occurs as plasma glucose levels decline within the physiological range. The secretion of glucose counterregulatory (plasma glucose–raising) hormones, including glucagon and epinephrine, increases as plasma glucose concentrations fall just below the postabsorptive physiological range. Lower glucose levels cause symptoms. Even lower levels cause functional brain failure (Cryer 2007). Prolonged, very low levels can cause brain death (Cryer 2007).

**Table 2.1.** Physiological Responses to
Decreasing Plasma Glucose Concentrations

| Response | Glycemic threshold* [mg/dl (mmol/l)] | Physiological effects | Role in prevention or correction of hypoglycemia (glucose counterregulation) |
|---|---|---|---|
| ↓ Insulin | 80–85 (4.4–4.7) | ↑$R_a$ (↓$R_d$) | Primary glucose regulatory factor, first defense against hypoglycemia |
| ↑ Glucagon | 65–70 (3.6–3.9) | ↑$R_a$ | Primary glucose counterregulatory factor, second defense against hypoglycemia |
| ↑ Epinephrine | 65–70 (3.6–3.9) | ↑$R_a$, ↓$R_d$ | Involved, critical when glucagon is deficient, third defense against hypoglycemia |
| ↑ Cortisol and growth hormone | 65–70 (3.6–3.9) | ↑$R_a$, ↓$R_d$ | Involved, not critical |
| Symptoms | 50–55 (2.8–3.1) | ↑Exogenous glucose | Prompt behavioral defense (food ingestion) |
| ↓ Cognition | <50 (<2.8) | — | Compromises behavioral defense |

*Arterialized venous, not venous, plasma glucose concentrations. $R_a$, rate of glucose appearance, glucose production by the liver and kidneys; $R_d$, rate of glucose disappearance, glucose utilization by insulin-sensitive tissues such as skeletal muscle (no direct effect on central nervous system glucose utilization).

## CLINICAL MANIFESTATIONS OF HYPOGLYCEMIA

Symptoms and signs of hypoglycemia are not specific (Towler et al. 1993). Thus, hypoglycemia is documented most convincingly by Whipple's triad (Whipple 1938): symptoms, signs, or both consistent with hypoglycemia, a low measured plasma glucose concentration, and resolution of those symptoms and signs after the plasma glucose level is raised (Cryer 2008). A requirement for formal documentation of Whipple's triad—including a laboratory measurement of a low plasma glucose concentration—is important for the initial demonstration that a hypoglycemic disorder exists in patients without diabetes, since such disorders are rare (Cryer 2008; Cryer et al. In press). On the other hand, in patients with diabetes treated with an insulin secretagogue or insulin, the likelihood that a given symptomatic episode is the result of hypoglycemia is high (Chapter 1). Ideally, such patients should always estimate their plasma glucose concentrations with a monitor when they suspect their glucose level is low. In reality, that is sometimes not practical and is often not done. Nonetheless, it could be reasoned that the detrimental effects of brief erroneous treatment for suspected hypoglycemia are less than those of failure to treat an episode of bona fide hypoglycemia (Cryer 2007).

## Symptoms

Symptoms of hypoglycemia are categorized as neuroglycopenic—those that are the direct result of brain glucose deprivation per se—and neurogenic (or autonomic)—those that are largely the result of the perception of physiological changes caused by the central nervous system (CNS)–mediated sympathoadrenal discharge triggered by hypoglycemia (Cryer 2007, 2008; Schwartz et al. 1987; Mitrakou et al. 1991; Fanelli et al. 1994a; Towler et al. 1993; DeRosa and Cryer 2004) (Figure 2.1 and Table 2.1). (There is a semantic issue here. Neurogenic symptoms are initiated by glucose deprivation at peripheral and central sensors, i.e., by neuroglycopenia. However, their generation includes activation of sympathoadrenal outflow from the brain through the spinal cord to preganglionic neurons innervating the adrenal medullae and sympathetic postganglionic neurons, and they are largely sympathetic neural in origin [DeRosa and Cryer 2004].)

Neuroglycopenic manifestations of hypoglycemia include cognitive impairments, behavioral changes, and psychomotor abnormalities, and, at lower plasma glucose levels, seizure and coma—all examples of functional brain failure (Cryer 2007). Ultimately, after profound, prolonged hypoglycemia, they include brain death (Cryer 2007).

Neurogenic manifestations of hypoglycemia include both adrenergic and cholinergic symptoms (Towler et al. 1993). These are largely the result of sympathetic neural rather than adrenomedullary activation, since bilaterally adrenalectomized individuals experience typical neurogenic symptoms (DeRosa and Cryer 2004). Adrenergic symptoms—mediated largely by norepinephrine released from sympathetic postganglionic neurons but perhaps also to some extent by circulating epinephrine released from the adrenal medullae—include palpitations, tremor, and anxiety/arousal (Towler et al. 1993; DeRosa and Cryer 2004). Cholinergic symptoms—mediated largely by acetylcholine released from sympathetic postganglionic neurons— include sweating, hunger, and paresthesias (Towler et al. 1993; DeRosa and Cryer 2004). This classification is based on the effects of adrenergic and cholinergic antagonists (Towler et al. 1993). To the extent that those enter the brain, some of these symptoms (e.g., anxiety/arousal and hunger [Schultes et al. 2003]) may be mediated through central as well as peripheral mechanisms. Principal components analysis leads to a somewhat different classification of the symptoms of hypoglycemia (McCrimmon et al. 2003a).

Awareness of hypoglycemia is largely the result of the perception of neurogenic symptoms (Towler et al. 1993). Thus, it follows that hypoglycemia unawareness in people with diabetes (Chapter 3) is largely the result of reduced sympathetic neural, rather than adrenomedullary, activation during hypoglycemia.

## Signs

Pallor and diaphoresis (caused by adrenergic cutaneous vasoconstriction and cholinergic stimulation of sweat glands, respectively) are common signs of hypoglycemia. Heart rate and systolic blood pressure are raised, but usually not greatly. Neuroglycopenic manifestations are often observable. Transient neurological deficits sometimes occur.

## SYSTEMIC GLUCOSE BALANCE

Normally, rates of glucose flux into and out of the circulation are coordinately regulated such that systemic glucose balance is maintained, hypoglycemia (as well as hyperglycemia) is prevented, and a continuous supply of glucose to the brain is assured (Cryer 2001, 2008) (Table 2.2). Glucose influx into the circulation is the sum of intermittent exogenous glucose delivery from ingested carbohydrates and regulated endogenous glucose production from the liver (and the kidneys). Glucose efflux out of the circulation is the sum of ongoing fixed glucose utilization, largely by the brain, but to a small extent by strictly

**Table 2.2.** Systemic Glucose Balance

| Glucose flux into the circulation | Glucose flux out of the circulation |
|---|---|
| Intermittent exogenous glucose delivery | Ongoing glucose utilization, largely by the brain (plus strictly glycolytic tissues) |
| + | + |
| Regulated endogenous glucose production:<br>• Liver: glycogenolysis and gluconeogenesis[1,3,4]<br>• Kidneys: gluconeogenesis[1,4] | Regulated glucose utilization:<br>• Muscle, fat, liver, kidneys, etc.[2,5] |

[1]Decreased by insulin; [2]increased by insulin; [3]increased by glucagon; [4]increased by epinephrine; [5]decreased by epinephrine.

glycolytic tissues such as the renal medullae and erythrocytes, and regulated glucose utilization by tissues such as muscle, fat, liver, and kidneys among others. Because exogenous glucose delivery is intermittent and more than half of glucose utilization (that by the brain) is fixed, systemic glucose balance is fine-tuned, and the plasma glucose concentration is maintained, by regulated endogenous glucose production and regulated glucose utilization by non-neural tissues (Cryer 2001, 2008; Cherrington 2001). Although an array of hormonal, neural, and substrate factors are involved, glucose production and utilization are regulated primarily by the pancreatic β-cell hormone insulin. As plasma glucose concentrations rise (e.g., after a meal), insulin secretion increases and both suppresses hepatic (and renal) glucose production and stimulates glucose utilization by muscle and fat. As plasma glucose concentrations decline (e.g., between meals), insulin secretion decreases and both increases hepatic (and renal) glucose production and decreases glucose utilization by muscle and fat. Importantly, although insulin does act on regions of the brain—to improve memory (Craft et al. 1996; Kern et al. 2001; Benedict et al. 2004, 2007), decrease appetite (Porte et al. 2005), activate parasympathetic inhibition of endogenous glucose production (Obici et al. 2002), and modulate regional glucose metabolism (Bingham et al. 2002), among other effects (Benedict et al. 2006)—it does not stimulate blood-to-brain glucose transport (Knudsen et al. 1999; Seaquist et al. 2001).

Insulin is a potent and critical hormone. Its deficiency causes hyperglycemia (diabetes), and its excess can cause hypoglycemia (Cryer 2001, 2008; Cherrington 2001). Nonetheless, it is not the only factor involved in maintenance of systemic glucose balance.

## GLUCOREGULATORY FACTORS

## Insulin

Insulin secretion is stimulated by glucose, amino acids, non-esterified fatty acids, $\beta_2$-adrenergic activation by catecholamines such as epinephrine, and acetylcholine released from parasympathetic nerves; it is inhibited by low glucose, $\alpha_2$-adrenergic activation by catecholamines such as norepinephrine released from sympathetic nerves, and somatostatin. Insulin secretion is very sensitive to fluctuations in the plasma glucose concentration within the physiological range (Cryer 2001, 2008; Cherrington 2001) (Table 2.1).

Insulin is secreted from pancreatic islet $\beta$-cells into the hepatic portal vein. Approximately 50% is extracted by the liver (Cherrington 2001). Insulin secretion can be quantified by measurements of the plasma concentrations of C-peptide, the peptide cleaved from proinsulin to produce insulin (Eaton et al. 1980; Polonsky et al. 1986). C-peptide is co-secreted with insulin but not cleared by the liver. Insulin secretion so calculated virtually ceases during hypoglycemia in humans (Heller and Cryer 1991a).

Insulin suppresses hepatic glycogenolysis rapidly and hepatic (and renal) gluconeogenesis more gradually and thus suppresses endogenous glucose production (Cryer 2001, 2008; Cherrington 2001; Edgerton et al. 2006). Basal insulin levels restrain glucose production in the postabsorptive state, and increased insulin levels suppress glucose production and stimulate glucose utilization in the postprandial state. The actions of insulin to suppress glucose production are both direct (via hepatic and renal insulin receptors) and indirect (Cryer 2001, 2008; Cherrington 2001; Obici et al. 2002; Edgerton et al. 2006; Bergman

2007). The hormone acts indirectly by inhibition of lipolysis, suppression of glucagon secretion, limitation of gluconeogenic precursor (e.g., amino acids, glycerol) flux from muscle and fat to the liver (and kidneys), and CNS-mediated activation of parasympathetic outflow.

Conversely, a decrease in insulin, as during decreasing plasma glucose concentrations and hypoglycemia, causes an increase in hepatic (and renal) glucose production, again initially an increase in hepatic glycogenolysis, and virtual cessation of glucose utilization by insulin-sensitive tissues (Cryer 2001, 2008; Cherrington 2001; Heller and Cryer 1991a). As discussed later in this chapter, a decrease in insulin is the first physiological defense against hypoglycemia (Cryer 2001, 2008).

## Glucagon

Glucagon secretion is stimulated by low glucose, amino acids, $\beta_2$-adrenergic activation by catecholamines such as epinephrine and norepinephrine, and acetylcholine released from parasympathetic nerves; it is inhibited by high glucose, insulin, nonesterified fatty acids, and somatostatin (Cryer 2001, 2008; Cherrington 2001). Whereas it is less sensitive to decreasing glucose levels than insulin secretion, glucagon secretion increases as plasma glucose concentrations fall just below the physiological range (Schwartz et al. 1987; Mitrakou et al. 1991; Fanelli et al. 1994a; Cherrington 2001) (Table 2.1). Glucagon secretion is regulated by both CNS-mediated and CNS-independent mechanisms (Cryer 2001, 2008; Cherrington 2001; Raju and Cryer 2005). CNS-mediated autonomic nervous system (sympathetic neural, parasympathetic neural, and adrenomedullary) activation increases glucagon secretion (Taborsky et al. 1998). However, low-glucose concentrations suppress insulin secretion and stimulate glucagon secretion in the absence of CNS signals, e.g., in spinal cord transected humans, from the transplanted human pancreas and the denervated dog pancreas, as well as from the isolated perfused pancreas and perifused pancreatic islets (Cryer 2001, 2008; Raju and Cryer 2005). Indeed, a decrease in intra-islet insulin, perhaps among other β-cell secretory products, signals an increase in glucagon secretion during hypoglycemia in humans (Raju and Cryer 2005).

Glucagon is secreted from pancreatic islet α-cells into the hepatic portal vein. Approximately 25% is extracted by the liver (Cherrington 2001). The hormone is thought to act only on the liver. The absence of a marker of glucagon secretion (analogous to C-peptide for insulin secretion) complicates the assessment of glucagon secretion in humans. Furthermore, available glucagon immunoassays measure species in addition to biologically active 3,500-Dalton glucagon, although changes in measured glucagon levels are thought to reflect changes in 3,500-Dalton glucagon (Cherrington 2001). In addition, because insulin suppresses glucagon secretion, the glucagon responses to hypoglycemia measured during contemporary hyperinsulinemic-hypoglycemic clamps are much less robust than the responses measured during hypoglycemia induced by an intravenous bolus injection of insulin.

Glucagon rapidly stimulates hepatic (but not renal) glucose production, largely by stimulating glycogenolysis (Cryer 2001, 2008; Cherrington 2001). The increase in glucose production and the plasma glucose concentration is transient, in part because of increased insulin secretion and the suppressive effect of hyperglycemia on glucose production (Cherrington 2001). Glucagon also stimulates hepatic gluconeogenesis when gluconeogenic precursors are abundant (Gustavson et al. 2003).

Glucagon, in concert with insulin, supports the postabsorptive plasma glucose concentration in humans (Cherrington 2001; Breckenridge et al. 2007). As discussed later in this chapter, an increase in glucagon is the second physiological defense against hypoglycemia (Cryer 2001, 2008).

## Epinephrine and the sympathoadrenal system

The autonomic nervous system includes the sympathetic nervous system and the adrenal medullae, collectively termed the sympathoadrenal system, and the parasympathetic nervous system. All three components are involved in metabolic regulation, including glucoregulation (Cryer 2001, 2008): sympathoadrenal activation raises plasma glucose concentrations and parasympathetic activation tends to lower plasma glucose concentrations. Postganglionic sympathetic neurons release norepinephrine or acetylcholine, and postganglionic parasympathetic neurons release acetylcholine, within innervated tissues. Whereas some extra-adrenal chromaffin cells persist into adult life, the major residual clusters of chromaffin cells comprise the adrenal medullae, which are virtually the sole source of the circulating hormone epinephrine (Cryer 2001, 2008; DeRosa and Cryer 2004). The anatomical relationship between the adrenal medullae and the adrenal cortices is important physiologically, since a portal venous system provides cortisol from the cortex to the medulla, where the enzyme that catalyzes the conversion of norepinephrine to epinephrine (phenylethanolamine-$N$-methyltransferase) is cortisol induced (Wurtman and Axelrod 1965; Wurtman 2002). Thus, adrenocortical cortisol deficiency results in adrenomedullary epinephrine deficiency (Wurtman 2002; Davis et al. 1997a), including a markedly reduced plasma epinephrine response to hypoglycemia in humans (Davis et al. 1997a).

Unlike insulin and glucagon secretion, which are regulated primarily by changes in glucose concentrations within the pancreatic islets and only secondarily by autonomic mechanisms, autonomic activity, including epinephrine secretion, is regulated within the CNS (Cryer 2001, 2008). For example, subphysiological plasma glucose concentrations, sensed in the periphery (e.g., in the portal and superior mesenteric veins) and in the CNS, trigger a centrally mediated sympathoadrenal discharge—the magnitude of which is a function of the nadir glucose concentration—resulting in an increase in circulating epinephrine and norepinephrine. The epinephrine response is derived almost exclusively from the adrenal medullae (DeRosa and Cryer 2004). Whereas circulating norepinephrine is largely derived from sympathetic nerves under resting and many stimulated (e.g., exercise) conditions, the increment in plasma norepinephrine during hypoglycemia is largely derived from the adrenal medullae (DeRosa and Cryer 2004).

The biochemistry and the integrated physiology of the human sympathoadrenal system have been reviewed in detail (Eisenhofer et al. 2004). Epinephrine and norepinephrine are released from adrenomedullary chromaffin cells into the circulation; as such, these catecholamines function as classical hormones (Cryer 2001, 2008). In addition, norepinephrine is released from axon terminals of sympathetic postganglionic neurons into synaptic clefts in direct relationship to adrenergic receptors on target cells and functions as a neurotransmitter (Cryer 2001, 2008). Most of the neurally released norepinephrine is recaptured into axon terminals (or is metabolized locally); perhaps only 10% enters the circulation (Cryer 2001, 2008). Most metabolism of catecholamines occurs in the cytoplasm of the cells in which the amines are produced as a result of leakage from storage vesicles into the cytoplasm or during transit through the cytoplasm after reuptake from the extracellular space (Eisenhofer et al. 2004). Sympathetic postganglionic neurons express the degradative enzyme monoamine oxidase and therefore produce deaminated metabolites of norepinephrine (e.g., 3,4-dihydroxyphenylglycol). However, adrenomedullary chromaffin cells also express the enzyme catechol-$O$-methyltransferase and produce primarily the 3-$O$-methyl metabolites of epinephrine and norepinephrine, metanephrine and normetanephrine (Eisenhofer et al. 2004). In humans, >90% of circulating metanephrine, and ~33% of circulating normetanephrine, is derived from the adrenal medullae (Eisenhofer et al. 2004). Thus, stimulated plasma metanephrine concentrations can be conceptualized as a measure of the adrenomedullary epinephrine secretory capacity.

Measurement of the plasma epinephrine concentration provides a useful index of adrenomedullary activity (DeRosa and Cryer 2004), although, like that of other hormones, it represents the balance between secretion and clearance. The evaluation of sympathetic neural activity is more problematic. Although circulating norepinephrine is largely derived from adrenergic sympathetic postganglionic neurons under resting and many stimulated conditions, the increase in plasma norepinephrine concentrations during hypoglycemia is largely derived from the adrenal medulla (DeRosa and Cryer 2004). Furthermore, even under the appropriate conditions, circulating norepinephrine represents only a small fraction of that released from sympathetic nerves and is the net result of differentiated regional nerve firing. Isotope dilution estimates of systemic and regional norepinephrine spillover have been used to overcome these shortcomings (Eisenhofer 2005; Paramore et al. 1998) and have documented sympathetic neural responses to hypoglycemia, although its fundamental assumptions have been questioned (Christensen and Norsk 2005). Microneurography measures muscle sympathetic nerve activity directly and has documented an increase in this nerve activity during hypoglycemia (Vallbo et al. 2004; Fagius 2003). However, the method is operator dependent, time-consuming, and demanding for the subject; does not allow movement by the subject; is not practical in the presence of autonomic neuropathy; and measures only one aspect of sympathetic nerve activity in only one region of the body (typically the lower extremity). Another approach is measurement of the extracellular norepinephrine concentration by microdialysis (Bruce et al. 2002; Maggs et al. 1997). That method has been used to document norepinephrine release in skeletal muscle and fat during hypoglycemia (Maggs et al. 1997). It requires careful calibration and is applicable to limited regions of the body. Finally, as noted earlier, adrenergic and cholinergic symptoms (Towler et al. 1993) reflect the sympathetic neural response to hypoglycemia (DeRosa an Cryer 2004).

Like glucagon, epinephrine rapidly stimulates hepatic glycogenolysis; it stimulates hepatic gluconeogenesis more prominently than glucagon (Gustavson et al. 2003). Unlike glucagon, epinephrine also stimulates renal gluconeogenesis and glucose production, limits glucose clearance by insulin-sensitive tissues such as muscle, mobilizes gluconeogenic precursors from muscle (lactate, amino acids) and fat (glycerol) to the liver and kidneys, and suppresses insulin secretion (Cryer 2001, 2008; Gustavson et al. 2003; Rizza et al. 1980; Berk et al. 1985).

The mechanisms of the plasma glucose–raising effect of epinephrine, summarized in Figure 2.2, are complex (Cryer 1993, 2001). They involve both direct (on the liver and kidneys) and

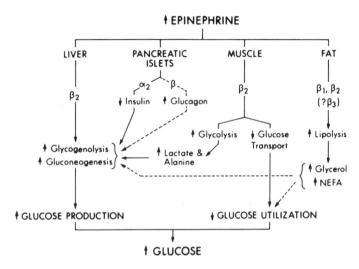

**Figure 2.2.** Mechanisms of the hyperglycemic effect of epinephrine. The α and β symbols refer to α-adrenergic and β-adrenergic receptors. From Cryer 1993, with permission from the American Diabetes Association.

indirect (other hormone- or substrate-mediated) actions, include both stimulation of glucose production and limitation of glucose utilization, and are mediated through both β- and α-adrenergic receptors. Whereas many of the actions of the hormone involve β2-adrenergic receptors (Figure 2.2), β-adrenergic activation alone has little plasma glucose–raising effect in healthy individuals because it stimulates insulin secretion. Thus, α2-adrenergic limitation of insulin secretion is normally an important aspect of the glycemic effect of epinephrine. Nonetheless, there is normally a small increase in insulin secretion—in response to β2-adrenergic β-cell stimulation, rising plasma glucose concentrations, or both—over time (Berk et al. 1985). That, too, is a critical glucoregulatory event because it limits the magnitude of the glycemic response. The glycemic response to epinephrine is increased substantially when insulin secretion is held constant pharmacologically in healthy individuals and in patients with type 1 diabetes who cannot increase insulin secretion (Berk et al. 1985). As discussed later in this chapter, an increase in epinephrine is the third defense against hypoglycemia.

Similar mechanisms are thought to be involved in the glycemic response to sympathetic neural norepinephrine release (Cryer 2001, 2008). The adrenergic and cholinergic neurogenic symptoms caused by the intense sympathoadrenal response to frank hypoglycemia prompt awareness of hypoglycemia (Towler et al. 1993; DeRosa and Cryer 2004). As discussed later in this chapter, that awareness prompts the behavioral defense against hypoglycemia.

## Cortisol and growth hormone

The plasma glucose–raising actions of glucagon and epinephrine occur within minutes (Cryer 2001, 2008; Cherrington 2001). In contrast, those of cortisol (Rizza et al. 1982) and growth hormone (MacGorman et al. 1981) (both of which support glucose production and limit glucose clearance) are delayed for several hours. Importantly, none of these hormones (glucagon, epinephrine, cortisol, or growth hormone) alters glucose transport across the blood-brain barrier.

## GLUCOSE COUNTERREGULATION: THE PREVENTION AND CORRECTION OF HYPOGLYCEMIA

## Physiological defenses

As reviewed in detail (Cryer 2001), there are three principles for the physiological prevention or correction of hypoglycemia

**Table 2.3.** Principles of Glucose Counterregulation in Humans

1. The prevention and correction of hypoglycemia are the result of both waning of insulin and activation of glucose counterregulatory systems. They are not due solely to waning of insulin.

2. Whereas insulin is the dominant plasma glucose–lowering factor, there are redundant glucose counterregulatory factors. Those include other hormones as well as substrates and perhaps neural factors.

3. There is a hierarchy among the glucoregulatory factors. Decrements in insulin, increments in glucagon, and, absent the latter, increments in epinephrine stand high in that hierarchy.

(Garber et al. 1976; Clarke et al. 1979; Gerich et al. 1979; Rizza et al. 1979) (Table 2.3). First, the prevention and correction of hypoglycemia are the result of both waning of insulin and activation of glucose counterregulatory (plasma glucose–raising) systems. They are not due solely to waning of insulin. After intravenous insulin injection, the changes in glucose kinetics that ultimately restore euglycemia begin while plasma insulin concentrations are still 10-fold above baseline and in temporal relation to increments in the plasma levels of counterregulatory hormones (Garber et al. 1976; Clarke et al. 1979). Similarly, the changes in glucose kinetics that limit the hypoglycemic response to prolonged hyperinsulinemia occur despite sustained hyperinsulinemia (De Feo et al. 1986). In addition, hypoinsulinemia is not critical to recovery from hypoglycemia (Heller and Cryer 1991a). Furthermore, when insulin levels are held constant, interruption of the secretion or actions of glucose counterregulatory factors impairs the prevention or correction of hypoglycemia (see following). Second, whereas insulin is the dominant plasma glucose–lowering factor, there are redundant glucose counterregulatory factors (Gerich et al. 1979; Rizza et al. 1979). These collectively constitute a fail-safe system that prevents or

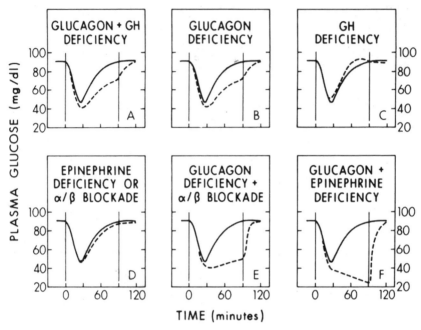

**Figure 2.3.** Summary of studies of the mechanisms of recovery from short-term hypoglycemia, induced by intravenous insulin injection at time 0 minutes, in humans. Interventions were started at time 0 minutes and stopped at time 90 minutes (i.e., between the vertical lines in each panel). Plasma glucose curves in control studies are indicated by the solid lines (the same in all panels), and plasma glucose curves under the indicated conditions are shown by the dashed lines. GH, growth hormone. From Cryer 1981, with permission from the American Diabetes Association.

minimizes failure of the glucose counterregulatory process upon failure of one, or perhaps more, of its components. Third, there is a hierarchy among the glucoregulatory factors, i.e., a ranked series of counterregulatory factors, some more critical to the effectiveness of the fail-safe system than others, that act in concert with decrements in insulin to prevent or correct hypoglycemia (Gerich et al. 1979; Rizza et al. 1979). Several aspects of this physiology are also shown in Table 2.1. Studies

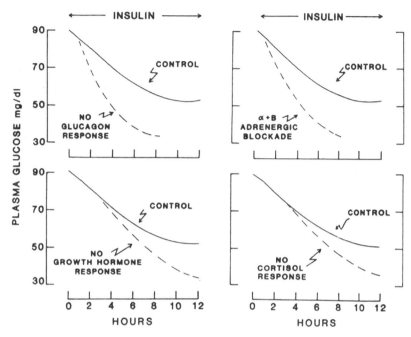

**Figure 2.4.** Summary of studies of the mechanisms of defense against prolonged insulin-induced hypoglycemia in humans. Plasma glucose curves in control studies are indicated by the solid lines (the same in all panels), and plasma glucose curves under the indicated conditions are shown by the dashed lines. From Gerich 1988, with permission from the American Diabetes Association.

of its mechanisms in humans are summarized in Figure 2.3 (Cryer 1981) and Figure 2.4 (Gerich 1988).

In defense against falling plasma glucose concentrations, decrements in insulin are fundamentally important. Insulin secretion virtually ceases during hypoglycemia and increments in insulin from suppressed levels impair recovery from hypoglycemia in a dose-related fashion (Heller and Cryer 1991a). An increase in insulin secretion is the first, and for practical purposes the only, defense against rising plasma glucose concentrations; loss of β-cell insulin secretion causes hyperglycemia (diabetes mellitus) and is fatal if insulin is not replaced. Conversely, a decrease in insulin secretion is the first, and arguably the most important, defense against falling plasma glucose concentrations. But, it is not the only defense. Glucose counterregulatory systems can prevent or correct hypoglycemia despite moderate hyperinsulinemia.

Among the glucose counterregulatory factors, glucagon plays a primary role (Gerich et al. 1979; Rizza et al. 1979). Albeit demonstrably involved, epinephrine is not normally critical. But, it becomes critical when glucagon is deficient. Isolated deficiency of the glucagon response (De Feo et al. 1991a) or of epinephrine actions (De Feo et al. 1991b) results in lower nadir plasma glucose concentrations early in the course of prolonged hypoglycemia. These data document that both glucagon and epinephrine are involved in defense against hyperinsulinemia. They do not address the relative roles of glucagon or epinephrine in the prevention or correction of hypoglycemia. Suppression of glucagon secretion (with somatostatin) impairs, but does not prevent, recovery from short-term hypoglycemia (Gerich et al. 1979; Rizza et al. 1979). That effect is reversed by glucagon, but not by growth hormone, replacement. In contrast, neither pharmacological adrenergic blockade nor epinephrine deficiency (bilateral adrenalectomy) impairs recovery from short-term hypoglycemia. However, progressive hypoglycemia develops when both glucagon and epinephrine are deficient. These data indicate that glucagon is involved in the correction of hypoglycemia, whereas epinephrine is not critical when glucagon secretion is intact. However, epinephrine becomes critical when glucagon secretion is deficient. Although progressive hypoglycemia does not develop, suppression of glucagon secretion lowers plasma glucose concentrations after an overnight fast (Breckenridge et al. 2007; Rosen et al. 1984), during a prolonged fast (Boyle et al. 1989), late after glucose ingestion (Tse et al. 1983a, 1983b), and during moderate exercise (Hirsch et al. 1991; Marker et al. 1991). In contrast, with the exception of a small effect during exercise, neither pharmacological adrenergic blockade nor epinephrine deficiency lowers plasma glucose concentrations under any of these conditions (Rosen et al. 1984; Boyle et al. 1989; Tse et al. 1983a, 1983b; Hirsch et al. 1991; Marker et al. 1991). However, combined glucagon deficiency and adrenergic blockade (or epinephrine deficiency) results in progressive hypoglycemia under all four conditions (Rosen et al. 1984; Boyle et al. 1989; Tse et al. 1983a, 1983b; Hirsch et al. 1991; Marker et al. 1991). These data further indicate that glucagon plays a role in the prevention and correction of hypoglycemia under diverse physiological conditions, whereas epinephrine is not critical when glucagon secretion is intact. However, epinephrine becomes critical to the prevention or correction of hypoglycemia under diverse conditions when glucagon secretion is deficient.

Growth hormone and cortisol stand lower in the hierarchy of physiological glucose counterregulatory factors than insulin, glucagon, and epinephrine (De Feo et al. 1989a, 1989b; Boyle and Cryer 1991). Both growth hormone (De Feo et al. 1989a) and cortisol (De Feo et al. 1989b) are involved in defense against prolonged hypoglycemia, but neither is critical to the correction of even prolonged hypoglycemia or the prevention of hypoglycemia after an overnight fast (Boyle and Cryer 1991).

There is evidence that glucose autoregulation—an increase in endogenous glucose production independent of hormonal and neural regulatory signals—is involved in glucose counter-regulation, albeit only during severe hypoglycemia (Bolli et al. 1985), and that nonesterified fatty acids mediate, at least in part, the glucose counterregulatory actions of epinephrine (Fanelli et al. 1992).

There is no clear evidence that efferent neural mechanisms normally play an important role in physiological glucose counterregulation. However, sympathoadrenal activation plays a key role in the behavioral defense against developing hypoglycemia.

## Behavioral defense

If the physiological defenses fail to reverse falling plasma glucose concentrations, lower plasma glucose levels trigger a more intense sympathoadrenal response, which causes symptoms (Towler et al. 1993; DeRosa and Cryer 2004) that allow the individual to recognize hypoglycemia. Again, the neurogenic symptoms of hypoglycemia are largely the result of sympathetic neural, rather than adrenomedullary, activation (DeRosa and Cryer 2004). That awareness of hypoglycemia prompts the behavioral defense against hypoglycemia, the ingestion of carbohydrates.

## INTEGRATED PHYSIOLOGY OF GLUCOSE COUNTERREGULATION

The integrated physiology of glucose counterregulation—the mechanisms that normally prevent or rapidly correct hypoglycemia in humans (Cryer 2001)—is summarized in Figure 2.5 (Cryer 2006b). The first defense against falling plasma glucose concentrations is a decease in pancreatic β-cell insulin secre-

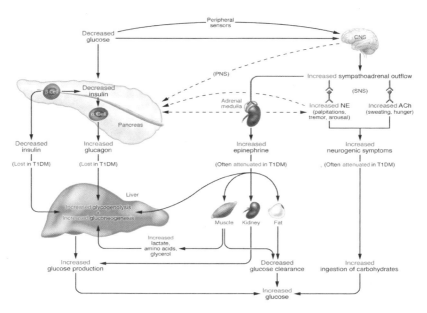

**Figure 2.5.** Physiological and behavioral defenses against hypoglycemia in humans. ACh, acetylcholine; NE, norepinephrine; PNS, parasympathetic nervous system; SNS, sympathetic nervous system; T1DM, type 1 diabetes. From Cryer 2006b, with permission from the American Society for Clinical Investigation.

tion. The second defense is an increase in pancreatic α-cell glucagon secretion. The third defense, which becomes critical when glucagon is deficient, is an increase in adrenomedullary epinephrine secretion. If these three physiological defenses fail to abort the episode, lower plasma glucose levels trigger a more intense sympathoadrenal (sympathetic neural as well as adrenomedullary) response that causes symptoms and thus awareness of hypoglycemia that prompts the behavioral defense.

The mechanisms of the normal responses to falling plasma glucose concentrations (Figure 2.5) are further illustrated in Figure 2.6. Low plasma glucose concentrations are sensed by

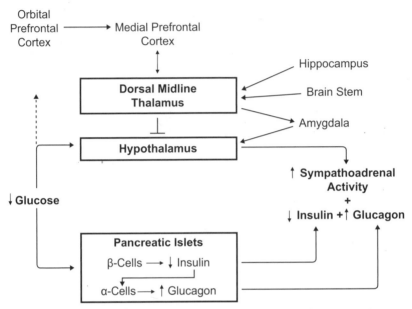

**Figure 2.6.** Schematic representation of the normal pancreatic, hypothalamic and cerebral mechanisms of the glucose counterregulatory responses to falling plasma glucose concentrations in humans.

pancreatic β-cells, resulting in a decrease in insulin secretion. The resulting decrease in intra-islet insulin, perhaps among other β-cell secretory products, in concert with low glucose levels, signals an increase in α-cell glucagon secretion (Raju and Cryer 2005). Thus, the first and second physiological defenses against falling plasma glucose concentrations—a decrement in insulin secretion and an increment in glucagon secretion—are mediated at the level of the pancreatic islets. Central nervous system (CNS) connections (i.e., innervation) are not required. Because appropriate changes in insulin and glucagon secretion are sufficient to accomplish defense against falling plasma glucose concentrations, the CNS is not normally critical to the prevention or correction of hypoglycemia. However, it becomes critical when the appropriate insulin and glucagon responses do not occur (Chapter 3).

Low plasma glucose concentrations are also sensed in peripheral sites (such as the portal and superior mesenteric veins) and transmitted to the brain and are sensed directly within the brain (Marty et al. 2007). There the hypothalamus initiates an increase in systemic sympathoadrenal activity, including the third physiological defense against falling plasma glucose concentrations—an increment in adrenomedullary epinephrine secretion. That increase in sympathoadrenal activity also includes activation of the sympathetic nervous system and thus, ultimately, the behavioral defense against falling plasma glucose concentrations (the ingestion of carbohydrates). While sympathoadrenal activation tends to decrease insulin secretion and increase glucagon secretion, those insulin and glucagon responses do not require a sympathoadrenal response, since they are also signaled at the level of the pancreatic islets (Raju and Cryer 2005).

There is increasing evidence that the hypothalamic response is modulated by widespread functionally interconnected cerebral inputs (Teves et al. 2004; Arbelaez et al. 2008), including an inhibitory pathway from the dorsal midline thalamus (Figure 2.6). However, the details of hypothalamic and cerebral mechanisms remain to be determined (Marty et al. 2007; McCrimmon 2008; Sherwin 2008).

At least in part because of the clinical importance of hypoglycemia in people with diabetes, studies of the molecular and cellular physiology and pathophysiology of the CNS-mediated neuroendocrine, including sympathoadrenal, responses to falling plasma glucose concentrations are an increasingly active area of fundamental neuroscience research. Some of these mechanisms have been reviewed (Marty et al. 2007; Cryer 2005; McCrimmon 2008; Sherwin 2008), and these are mentioned in the context of the pathophysiology of glucose counterregulation in diabetes in Chapter 3.

It is interesting that there is only one physiologically effective defense against hyperglycemia, the glucoregulatory hormone insulin, whereas there are redundant physiological and behavioral defenses against hypoglycemia. This may explain why glucoregulatory failure due to relative or absolute insulin deficiency causing hyperglycemia (diabetes mellitus) is common, whereas glucose counterregulatory failure causing hypoglycemia is rare in the absence of drug-treated diabetes. This dichotomy is plausibly explained by evolutionary pressure (Cryer 1997). Typically developing later in life, diabetes would have threatened survival of the individual. In contrast, hypoglycemia would have threatened survival of the species. The irony is that in the setting of demonstrably effective insulin secretagogue or insulin therapy of diabetes, the causative β-cell failure also leads to compromised physiological and behavioral defenses against hypoglycemia (Chapter 3).

# Chapter 3.
# The Pathophysiology of Glucose Counterregulation in Diabetes

## OVERVIEW: INTERPLAY OF INSULIN EXCESS AND COMPROMISED GLUCOSE COUNTERREGULATION

As developed in Chapter 1, iatrogenic hypoglycemia is the limiting factor in the glycemic management of diabetes (Cryer 2004, 2008). It causes recurrent morbidity in most people with type 1 diabetes and many with advanced type 2 diabetes and is sometimes fatal. In addition, it precludes maintenance of euglycemia over a lifetime of diabetes and thus full realization of the vascular benefits of long-term glycemic control. Furthermore, as discussed in this chapter, it compromises defenses against subsequent hypoglycemia and thus causes a vicious cycle of recurrent hypoglycemia.

Hypoglycemia in diabetes is typically the result of the interplay of relative or absolute therapeutic insulin excess and compromised defenses against falling plasma glucose concentrations (Cryer 2004, 2008). Thus, it is fundamentally iatrogenic, the result of treatments that raise circulating insulin levels and thus lower plasma glucose concentrations (Chapter 2). Those treatments include insulin and insulin secretagogues such as a sulfonylurea (e.g., glyburide [glibenclamide], glipizide, or glimepiride among others) or a non-sulfonylurea secretagogue (e.g., nateglinide, repaglinide). All people with type 1 diabetes must be treated with insulin. Most people with type 2 diabetes ultimately require treatment with insulin. Early in the course of the disease, individuals with type 2 diabetes may respond to treatment with an insulin secretagogue. Alternatively, they may respond to drugs that do not raise insulin levels, at least when plasma glucose concentrations fall into and below the physiological range. The latter include a biguanide (metformin), thiazolidinediones (e.g., pioglitazone, rosiglitazone), α-glucosidase inhibitors (e.g., acarbose, miglitol), glucagon-like peptide-1 receptor agonists (e.g., exenatide, liraglutide), and dipeptidyl peptidase-IV inhibitors (e.g., sitagliptin, vildagliptin). These drugs should not, and probably do not (Bolen 2007), cause hypoglycemia when used as monotherapy, although metformin has been reported to cause self-reported hypoglycemia (UKPDS 1995; Wright et al. 2006), or in combination among themselves (Chapter 1). However, they can increase the risk of hypoglycemia when used with insulin or with an insulin secretagogue (de Heer and Holst 2007).

## INSULIN EXCESS

Relative or even absolute insulin excess must occur from time to time during treatment with an insulin secretagogue or with insulin because of the pharmacokinetic imperfections of these therapies. Even the most sophisticated regimens do not replicate normal (endogenous) insulin secretion, which is plasma glucose regulated and during which variations in circulating insulin levels occur over minutes. With an insulin secretagogue or insulin, to the extent the patient has deficient endogenous insulin secretion, insulin levels are not plasma glucose regulated. Furthermore, variations in insulin levels occur over hours.

Insulin excess of sufficient magnitude can, of course, cause hypoglycemia. However, as developed in Chapter 1, the frequency of hypoglycemia is relatively low (at least with currently recommended glycemic goals), even during therapy with insulin early in the course of type 2 diabetes. (Indeed, it is relatively low very early in the course of type 1 diabetes—the "honeymoon" period.) Therefore, factors in addition to relative or absolute therapeutic insulin excess must play an important role in the pathogenesis of hypoglycemia, which becomes progressively more frequent over time—rapidly in type 1 diabetes and gradually in type 2 diabetes (Chapter 1). Those additional factors are progressive failure of the normal physiological and behavioral defenses against falling plasma glucose concentrations (Chapter 2). Thus, while therapeutic hyperinsulinemia, either relative (to low rates of exogenous or endogenous glucose flux into the circulation or high rates of glucose flux out of the circulation) or absolute, is a prerequisite for the development of hypoglycemia in diabetes, compromised glucose counterregulation is the key feature of the pathogenesis of iatrogenic hypoglycemia in type 1 diabetes and advanced type 2 diabetes (Cryer 2004, 2008).

## COMPROMISED GLUCOSE COUNTERREGULATION

As discussed in Chapter 2, the key physiological defenses against falling plasma glucose concentrations (Figure 2.5) include 1) decrements in pancreatic islet β-cell insulin secretion, 2) increments in pancreatic islet α-cell glucagon secretion, and, absent the latter, 3) increments in adrenomedullary epinephrine secretion (Cryer 2001, 2008). The behavioral defense is the ingestion of carbohydrates prompted by symptoms—largely sympathetic neural neurogenic symptoms (DeRosa and Cryer 2004)—that make the individual aware of hypoglycemia (Cryer 2001, 2008). All of these are typically compromised in type 1 diabetes and advanced type 2 diabetes (Cryer 2004, 2008; Dagogo-Jack et al. 1993; Segel et al. 2002).

In fully developed (i.e., C-peptide–negative) type 1 diabetes, circulating insulin levels do not decrease as plasma glucose concentrations decline through or below the physiological range. In the absence of functioning β-cells, plasma insulin levels are simply a passive function of the clearance of administered (exogenous) insulin. Furthermore, in the absence of a β-cell signal, a decrease in intra-islet insulin perhaps among others (Raju and Cryer 2005), circulating glucagon levels do not increase as plasma glucose concentrations fall below the physiological range (Gerich et al. 1973) (Figure 3.1). Thus, both the first defense against hypoglycemia—a decrease in insulin levels—and the second defense against hypoglycemia—an increase in glucagon levels—are lost in type 1 diabetes. Therefore, patients with type 1 diabetes are critically dependent on the third defense against hypoglycemia, an increase in epinephrine levels. However, the epinephrine secretory response to hypoglycemia is often attenuated in type 1 diabetes (Cryer 2004, 2008; Dagogo-Jack et al. 1993) (Figure 3.1). Through mechanisms yet to be clearly defined but often thought to reside in the brain (Cryer 2004, 2005, 2006, 2008), the glycemic threshold for sympathoadrenal—both adrenomedullary and sympathetic neural—activation is shifted to lower plasma glucose concentrations by recent antecedent hypoglycemia (Cryer 2004, 2005, 2006, 2008; Dagogo-Jack et al. 1993; Segel et al. 2002) (Figures 3.2 and 3.3), as well as by prior exercise (Cryer 2004, 2005,

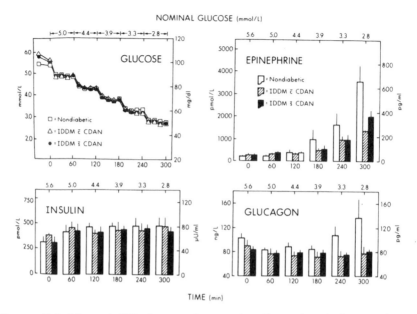

**Figure 3.1.** Mean (+SE) plasma glucose, insulin, epinephrine, and glucagon concentrations during hyperinsulinemic stepped hypoglycemia glucose clamps in nondiabetic individuals (open squares and columns), people with type 1 diabetes (IDDM, insulin dependent diabetes mellitus) with classical diabetic autonomic neuropathy (CDAN) (open triangles and cross-hatched columns), and people with type 1 diabetes without CDAN (closed circles and columns). From Dagogo-Jack et al. 1993, with permission from the American Society for Clinical Investigation.

2006, 2008; Galassetti et al. 2001; Sandoval et al. 2004; Ertl and Davis 2004) and by sleep (Cryer 2004, 2005, 2006, 2008; Jones et al. 1998; Banarer and Cryer 2003; Schultes et al. 2007).

The patterns of plasma insulin, glucagon, and epinephrine responses to falling plasma glucose concentrations in nondiabetic individuals, people with type 1 diabetes, and people with type 2 diabetes are summarized in Table 3.1. The reduced responses to a given level of hypoglycemia in people with diabetes cause the clinical syndromes of defective glucose coun-

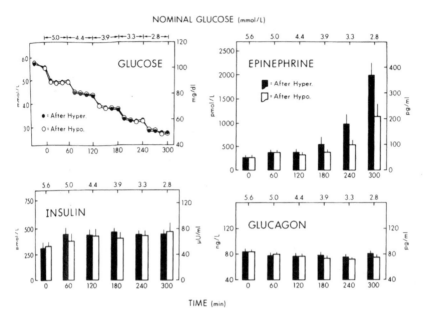

**Figure 3.2.** Mean (+SE) plasma glucose, insulin, epinephrine, and glucagon concentrations during hyperinsulinemic stepped hypoglycemic glucose clamps in patients with type 1 diabetes (IDDM, insulin dependent diabetes mellitus) without classical diabetic autonomic neuropathy on mornings following afternoon hyperglycemia (After Hyper., closed circles and columns) and on mornings following afternoon hypoglycemia (After Hypo., open circles and columns). From Dagogo-Jack et al. 1993, with permission from the American Society for Clinical Investigation.

terregulation and hypoglycemia unawareness (Cryer 2004, 2008).

## Defective glucose counterregulation

In the setting of absent decrements in insulin and absent increments in glucagon, attenuated increments in epinephrine as plasma glucose levels fall in response to therapeutic hyperinsulinemia cause the clinical syndrome of defective glucose counterregulation (Cryer 2004, 2008) (Table 3.1). Compared

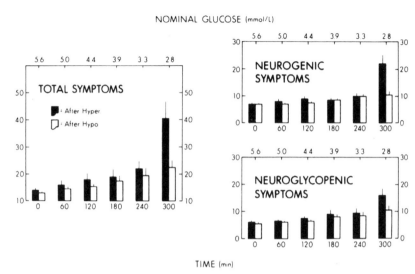

**Figure 3.3.** Mean (+SE) total, neurogenic, and neuroglycopenic symptom scores during hyperinsulinemic stepped hypoglycemic clamps in patients with type 1 diabetes (IDDM, insulin dependent diabetes mellitus) without classical diabetic autonomic neuropathy on mornings following afternoon hyperglycemia (After hyper., closed columns) and on mornings following afternoon hypoglycemia (After hypo., open columns). From Dagogo-Jack et al. 1993, with permission from the American Society for Clinical Investigation.

with patients with type 1 diabetes who also have absent insulin and glucagon responses but have normal epinephrine responses, patients with absent insulin and glucagon responses and reduced epinephrine responses have been shown to be at 25-fold (White et al. 1983) or greater (Bolli et al. 1984) increased risk for severe iatrogenic hypoglycemia during aggressive glycemic therapy. Originally identified by the failure of glycemic defense against low-dose insulin infusions (White et al. 1983; Bolli et al. 1984), the clinical syndrome of defective glucose counterregulation is characterized by absent decrements in insulin, absent increments in glucagon, and attenuated increments in epinephrine

**Table 3.1.** Responses to Falling Plasma Glucose Concentrations in Humans

| Plasma glucose | Individuals | -------------------------Plasma ------------------------- | | |
|---|---|---|---|---|
| — | | Insulin | Glucagon | Epinephrine |
| ↓ | Non-diabetic | ↓ | ↑ | ↑ |
| ↓ | Type 1 diabetes | No ↓ | No ↑ | Attenuated ↑ |
| | • Defective glucose counterregulation <br> • Hypoglycemia unawareness | | | |
| ↓ | Type 2 diabetes - Early | ↓ | ↑ | ↑ |
| ↓ | Type 2 diabetes - Late | No ↓ | No ↑ | Attenuated ↑ |

at a given level of hypoglycemia in insulin-deficient diabetes (Cryer 2004, 2008).

## Hypoglycemia unawareness

An attenuated epinephrine response to hypoglycemia (Table 3.1) is a marker of an attenuated sympathoadrenal—sympathetic neural as well as adrenomedullary—response. Largely as a result of an attenuated sympathetic neural response (DeRosa and Cryer 2004), the attenuated sympathoadrenal response causes the clinical syndrome of hypoglycemia unawareness (or impaired awareness of hypoglycemia)—impairment or even complete loss of the warning, largely neurogenic symptoms that previously prompted the behavioral defense, the ingestion of carbohydrates. Hypoglycemia unawareness is associated with a sixfold increased risk for severe hypoglycemia (Geddes et al. 2008).

It is generally thought that hypoglycemia unawareness is due to reduced release of the sympathetic neural neurotransmitters norepinephrine and acetylcholine and perhaps also that of adrenomedullary epinephrine (DeRosa and Cryer 2004). However, there is evidence of decreased β-adrenergic sensitivity, specifically reduced cardiac chronotropic sensitivity to isoproterenol (Berlin et al. 1987; Fritsche et al. 2001), in patients with unawareness. But vascular sensitivity to infusion of a β$_2$-adrenergic agonist was not found to be reduced in patients with unawareness (de Galan et al. 2006). Furthermore, reduced symptomatic β-adrenergic sensitivity remains to be demonstrated specifically in patients with unawareness. Finally, it would be necessary also to postulate reduced cholinergic sensitivity to explain reduced cholinergic symptoms such as sweating.

## HYPOGLYCEMIA-ASSOCIATED AUTONOMIC FAILURE

Based on the pivotal finding that a 2-hour episode of afternoon hypoglycemia, compared with afternoon euglycemia, reduced the sympathoadrenal and symptomatic (among other) responses to hypoglycemia the following morning in nondiabetic individuals (Heller and Cryer 1991b), the concept of hypoglycemia-associated autonomic failure (HAAF) in diabetes (Cryer 1992, 2004, 2005, 2006, 2008; Dagogo-Jack et al. 1993; Segel et al. 2002; Galassetti et al. 2001; Sandoval et al. 2004; Ertl and Davis 2004; Jones et al. 1998; Banarer and Cryer 2003; Schultes et al. 2007) was formulated (Cryer 1992) and then documented in patients with type 1 diabetes (Dagogo-Jack et al. 1993) and advanced type 2 diabetes (Segel et al. 2002).

The concept of HAAF in diabetes (Cryer 2004, 2008) posits that recent antecedent hypoglycemia (Dagogo-Jack et al. 1993; Segel et al. 2002; Cryer 2005, 2006b), as well as prior exercise (Galassetti et al. 2001; Sandoval et al. 2004; Ertl and Davis 2004) and sleep (Jones et al. 1998; Banarer and Cryer 2003; Schultes et al. 2007), causes both defective glucose counter-regulation (by reducing the adrenomedullary epinephrine response [Figure 3.2] in the absence of decrements in insulin and increments in glucagon) and hypoglycemia unawareness (by reducing the sympathoadrenal, including the sympathetic neural, and the resulting neurogenic symptom responses [Figure 3.3]) and therefore a vicious cycle of recurrent hypoglycemia. The concept of HAAF is illustrated in Figure 3.4.

HAAF is, at least in large part, a functional disorder distinct from classical diabetic autonomic neuropathy (Dagogo-Jack et al. 1993). It is a dynamic phenomenon that can be induced (by prior hypoglycemia or exercise or by sleep) and largely reversed (e.g., by avoidance of hypoglycemia) and is manifested clinically by recurrent iatrogenic hypoglycemia. In contrast, diabetic autonomic neuropathy is a structural disorder that is manifested clinically by gastrointestinal or genitourinary symptoms, by orthostatic hypotension, or by combinations of these and is not reversible. Nonetheless, there is evidence that the key feature of HAAF—an attenuated sympathoadrenal response to a given level of hypoglycemia—is more prominent in patients with diabetic autonomic neuropathy (Bottini et al. 1997; Meyer et al. 1998). That is illustrated in Figure 3.1 (Dagogo-Jack et al. 1993). Indeed, recent antecedent hypoglycemia reduces sympathoadrenal responses to subsequent hemodynamic stimuli, and reduces baroreflex sensitivity (Adler et al. In press). Thus, HAAF includes a form of autonomic failure functionally analo-

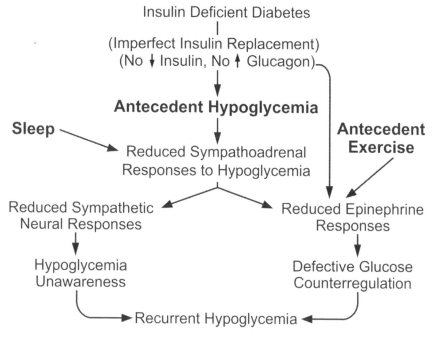

# Hypoglycemia-Associated Autonomic Failure

**Figure 3.4.** Schematic diagram of hypoglycemia-associated autonomic failure (HAAF) in diabetes. Modified from Cryer 2004, with permission from the Massachusetts Medical Society.

gous to autonomic neuropathy with respect to cardiovascular, as well as metabolic, regulation.

The clinical impact of HAAF is well established in type 1 diabetes (Dagogo-Jack et al. 1993, 1994; White et al. 1983; Bolli et al. 1984; Geddes et al. 2008; Fanelli et al. 1993, 1994b, 1998; Ovalle et al. 1998; Cranston et al. 1994). For example, recent antecedent hypoglycemia, even asymptomatic nocturnal hypoglycemia, reduces epinephrine, symptomatic, and cognitive dysfunction responses to a given level of subsequent hypoglycemia (Fanelli et al. 1998); reduces detection of hypoglycemia in the clinical setting (Ovalle et al. 1998); and reduces glycemic defense against hyperinsulinemia (Dagogo-Jack et al. 1993) in type 1 diabetes. Perhaps the most compelling support for the concept of HAAF is the finding, in three independent laboratories, that as little as 2–3 weeks of scrupulous avoidance of hypoglycemia reverses hypoglycemia unawareness (Figure 3.5) and improves the reduced epinephrine component of defective glucose counterregulation in most affected patients (Fanelli et al. 1993, 1994b; Cranston et al. 1994; Dagogo-Jack et al. 1994).

Developed initially in type 1 diabetes (Cryer 2004, 2008; Dagogo-Jack et al. 1993), the concept of HAAF has been extended to type 2 diabetes (Cryer 2004, 2008; Segel et al. 2002). In advanced (i.e., absolutely endogenous insulin–deficient) type 2 diabetes, glucagon responses to hypoglycemia are lost (Segel et al. 2002), as they are in type 1 diabetes. Furthermore, the glycemic thresholds for epinephrine and symptom responses (among other responses) are shifted to lower plasma glucose concentrations by recent antecedent hypoglycemia in type 2 diabetes (Segel et al. 2002), as they are in type 1 diabetes. Thus, people with advanced type 2 diabetes are also at risk for HAAF.

In summary, the pathophysiology of glucose counterregulation, and thus the pathogenesis of iatrogenic hypoglycemia, is basically the same in type 1 diabetes and type 2 diabetes. Iatrogenic hypoglycemia is typically the result of the interplay of therapeutic hyperinsulinemia and compromised defenses against falling plasma glucose concentrations (HAAF in diabetes). However, because HAAF stems fundamentally from β-cell failure (Cryer 2004, 2008; Raju and Cryer 2005), which results in loss of both the insulin and glucagon responses, setting the stage for the effect of attenuated sympathoadrenal responses to

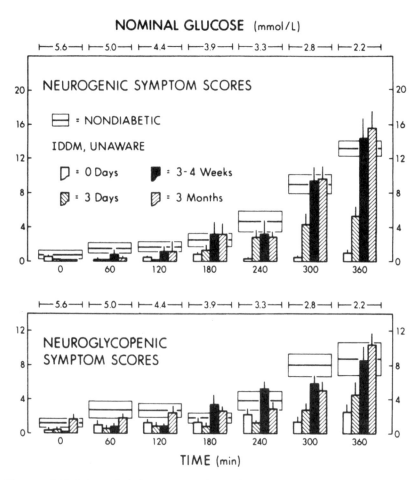

**Figure 3.5.** Mean (+SE) neurogenic and neuroglycopenic symptom scores during hyperinsulinemic stepped hypoglycemic clamps in non-diabetic individuals (rectangles) and in patients with type 1 diabetes (IDDM, columns) at baseline (0 days), after 3 days of inpatient strict avoidance of hypoglycemia, and after 3–4 weeks and 3 months of outpatient scrupulous avoidance of hypoglycemia. From Dagogo-Jack et al. 1994, with permission from the American Diabetes Association.

cause defective glucose counterregulation, as well as hypoglycemia unawareness, it develops rapidly in type 1 diabetes (in which β-cell failure develops rapidly) but slowly in type 2 diabetes (in which absolute β-cell failure develops slowly). That explains the relatively low frequency of hypoglycemia (at least with currently recommended glycemic goals) early in the course of type 2 diabetes and the relatively high frequency of hypoglycemia, approaching that in type 1 diabetes, as patients approach the insulin-deficient end of the spectrum of type 2 diabetes (Chapter 1).

## DIVERSE CAUSES OF HAAF

It is now recognized that there are diverse causes of HAAF in diabetes (Cryer 2004, 2008) (Figure 3.4). Those include 1) HAAF induced by recent antecedent iatrogenic hypoglycemia—hypoglycemia-related HAAF (Dagogo-Jack et al. 1993; Segel et al. 2002; Cryer 2005, 2006); 2) HAAF induced by prior exercise—exercise-related HAAF (Galassetti et al. 2001; Sandoval et al. 2004; Ertl and Davis 2004); and 3) HAAF induced by sleep—sleep-related HAAF (Jones et al. 1998; Banarer and Cryer 2003; Schultes et al. 2007) (Figure 3.4). Each of these inciting events causes reduced sympathoadrenal and symptomatic responses to a given level of subsequent hypoglycemia, the key feature of HAAF (i.e., sympathoadrenal failure associated with the development of iatrogenic hypoglycemia in diabetes). Indeed, it is conceivable that there are additional causes of HAAF.

### Hypoglycemia-related HAAF

Recent antecedent iatrogenic hypoglycemia was the first

recognized cause of HAAF and led to the concept (Cryer 2004, 2008; Dagogo-Jack et al. 1993; Segel et al. 2002; Cryer 2005, 2006) (Figure 3.5).

## Exercise-related HAAF

Moderate-intensity exercise increases glucose utilization (by exercising muscle) two- to threefold. In nondiabetic individuals, decrements in insulin, increments in glucagon, and, during intense exercise, increments in catecholamines result in increases in glucose production that generally match, or even exceed, those in glucose utilization, and hypoglycemia does not occur (Ertl and Davis 2004). However, largely because insulin levels are unregulated, hypoglycemia occurs commonly during or shortly after exercise in people with type 1 diabetes (Tansey et al. 2006).

While the risk of hypoglycemia during or shortly after exercise in type 1 diabetes is generally recognized, the risk of late post-exercise hypoglycemia (MacDonald 1987; Tsalikian et al. 2005) is less widely appreciated. Post-exercise late-onset hypoglycemia in type 1 diabetes, typically nocturnal and occurring 6–15 hours after unusually strenuous exercise, was nicely described by MacDonald more than two decades ago (MacDonald 1987). In one study, a quarter of patients with type 1 diabetes suffered nocturnal hypoglycemia in the absence of exercise the previous afternoon and half of the patients suffered nocturnal hypoglycemia after exercise the previous afternoon (Tsalikian et al. 2005). That follows directly from the pathophysiology of glucose counterregulation (Galassetti et al. 2001; Sandoval et al. 2004; Ertl and Davis 2004). Davis and colleagues have shown that exercise reduces sympathoadrenal responses to a given level of hypoglycemia several hours later in both nondiabetic individuals (Galassetti et al. 2001) and people with type 1 diabetes (Sandoval et al. 2004). The latter have absent insulin and glucagon responses and reduced sympathoadrenal and symptomatic responses to hypoglycemia, and their sympathoadrenal responses are reduced further after exercise (Sandoval et al. 2004). They have exercise-related HAAF (Cryer 2004, 2008; Ertl and Davis 2004) and therefore an increased risk of hypoglycemia (Tsalikian et al. 2005).

## Sleep-related HAAF

In people with type 1 diabetes, sympathoadrenal responses to a given level of hypoglycemia are reduced further during sleep (Jones et al. 1998; Banarer and Cryer 2003). Perhaps because of their further reduced sympathoadrenal responses, they are much less likely to be awakened by hypoglycemia than nondiabetic individuals (Banarer and Cryer 2003; Schultes et al. 2007). Thus, sleeping patients with type 1 diabetes have both further reduced epinephrine responses to hypoglycemia, the key feature of defective glucose counterregulation, and reduced arousal from sleep, a form of hypoglycemia unawareness. They have sleep-related HAAF (Cryer 2004, 2008; Jones et al. 1998; Banarer and Cryer 2003; Schultes et al. 2007) and are at high risk for hypoglycemia (Raju et al. 2006).

## Additional causes of HAAF

There may be as yet unrecognized functional, and thus potentially reversible, causes of HAAF in addition to recent antecedent hypoglycemia, prior exercise, and sleep. Furthermore, there may well be a structural factor, since the adrenal medullae can be conceptualized as postganglionic neurons without axons and therefore could be subject to neuropathy

(Dagogo-Jack et al. 1993; Bottini et al. 1997; Meyer et al. 1998). Indeed, there are clues to a fixed reduction of the epinephrine response to a given level of hypoglycemia in people with long-standing type 1 diabetes. First, while it reverses hypoglycemia unawareness, scrupulous avoidance of iatrogenic hypoglycemia improves but does not fully normalize the plasma epinephrine response to hypoglycemia (Fanelli et al. 1993, 1994b; Cranston et al. 1994; Dagogo-Jack et al. 1994). Second, when it is successful by producing insulin independence, islet transplantation virtually eliminates hypoglycemia and normalizes the glycemic threshold for epinephrine secretion and increases its magnitude, but it does not fully normalize the magnitude of the epinephrine response (Rickels et al. 2007). Third, as mentioned earlier, the epinephrine response to hypoglycemia is reduced to a greater extent in patients with clinically apparent classical diabetic autonomic neuropathy than it is in individuals without overt evidence of that complication (Bottini et al. 1997; Meyer et al. 1998). Fourth, the finding of a reduced plasma metanephrine, as well as epinephrine, response to hypoglycemia in patients with HAAF suggests a reduced adrenomedullary epinephrine secretory capacity (de Galan et al. 2004).

## MECHANISMS OF HAAF

HAAF develops in the setting of absent decrements in insulin and absent increments in glucagon as plasma glucose concentrations fall in response to therapeutic hyperinsulinemia in type 1 diabetes and advanced type 2 diabetes (Cryer 2004, 2008). The mechanisms of these prerequisite abnormalities are different from those of the attenuated sympathoadrenal and resulting symptomatic responses to hypoglycemia that ultimately cause the clinical syndromes of defective glucose counterregulation and hypoglycemia unawareness, the components of HAAF (Cryer 2004, 2008), as discussed earlier. These mechanisms are summarized in Figure 3.6.

## Absent insulin and glucagon responses

Because both type 1 diabetes and advanced (i.e., absolutely endogenous insulin–deficient) type 2 diabetes are the result of pancreatic islet β-cell failure, the mechanism of the loss of a decrement in insulin as plasma glucose concentrations decline within and below the physiological range is straightforward. That of the loss of the increment in glucagon is less clear-cut (Cryer 2004, 2005, 2008).

Glucagon secretory responses to stimuli other than hypoglycemia occur in patients with insulin-deficient diabetes who have no glucagon response to hypoglycemia (Wiethop and Cryer 1993a; Caprio et al. 1993; Hoffman et al. 1994). Therefore, loss of the glucagon response to falling plasma glucose concentrations in type 1 diabetes (Dagogo-Jack et al. 1993, 1994; Gerich et al. 1973; White et al. 1983; Fanelli et al. 1993, 1998; Ovalle et al. 1998; Bolli et al. 1983; Fukuda et al. 1988) and advanced type 2 diabetes (Segel et al. 2002) must be largely the result of a defect in signaling to functional glucagon secreting pancreatic islet α-cells.

Normally, there are redundant signals to glucagon-secretion during hypoglycemia. At least during marked hypoglycemia, which normally triggers an intense autonomic response, sympathetic neural, adrenomedullary, and parasympathetic neural signals stimulate glucagon secretion (Taborsky et al. 1998). However, adrenergic blockade does not prevent the glucagon response to hypoglycemia in humans (Rizza et al. 1979) and

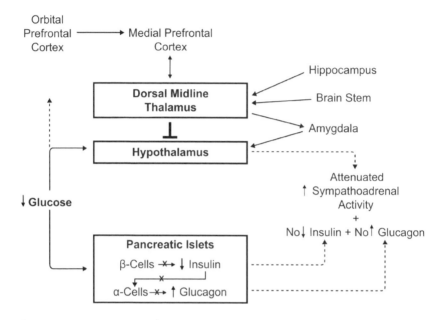

**Figure 3.6.** Pancreatic islet, hypothalamic, and cerebral network mechanisms of hypoglycemia-associated autonomic failure (HAAF) in diabetes. Compare with Figure 2.6.

epinephrine-deficient bilaterally adrenalectomized individuals have a normal glucagon response to hypoglycemia (DeRosa and Cryer 2004). Furthermore, neural signals are not critical to the insulin and glucagon responses to hypoglycemia. The denervated (i.e., transplanted) human pancreas (Diem et al. 1990) and the denervated dog pancreas (Sherck et al. 2001), as well as the perfused pancreas and perifused pancreatic islets, respond to low glucose levels with a decrease in insulin release and an increase in glucagon release (Figure 3.7). Therefore, loss of pancreatic sympathetic innervation (Mundinger et al. 2003) cannot explain loss of these responses to hypoglycemia in insulin-deficient diabetes, a conclusion consistent with the fact that loss of the glucagon response is not associated with clinical diabetic autonomic neuropathy in type 1 diabetes (Dagogo-Jack et al. 1993). On the other hand, the degree of loss of the glucagon response is associated with the degree of loss of insulin secretion (Fukuda et al. 1988). Therefore, loss of the glucagon response to hypoglycemia in insulin-deficient diabetes is the result of alterations of signaling within the diseased pancreatic islets rather than loss of extrinsic autonomic signaling to those islets (Figures 3.6 and 3.7).

First formulated by Samols et al. in 1972 and based on findings from the perfused rat pancreas (Maruyama et al. 1984; Samols et al. 1988)—including the finding that perfusion with an antibody to insulin causes increased glucagon release (Maruyama et al. 1984)—and later findings in rats in vivo (Zhou et

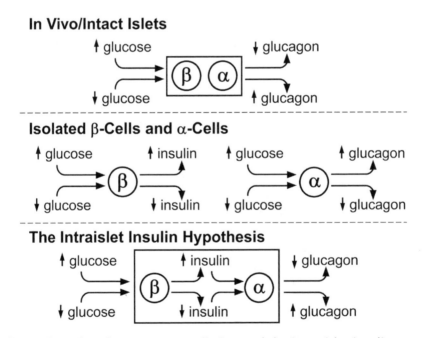

**Figure 3.7.** The glucagon contradiction and the intra-islet insulin hypothesis.

al. 2004) and isolated rat α-cells (Olsen et al. 2005; Gromada et al. 2007), the intra-islet insulin hypothesis posits that α-cell glucagon secretion is regulated reciprocally by β-cell insulin, perhaps along with other β-cell secretory products (Gromada et al. 2007; Zhou, Zhang et al. 2007), via the islet microcirculation (Figure 3.7). With respect to the glucagon response to hypoglycemia, the concept is that a low plasma glucose concentration acts on β-cells to cause a decrease in insulin secretion and thus a decrease in intra-islet insulin, which in turn reduces tonic inhibition of α-cell glucagon secretion by insulin, resulting in increased glucagon secretion during hypoglycemia (Figure 3.7).

The notion that α-cell glucagon secretion is regulated indirectly by a glucose-modulated β-cell secretory product or products has been endorsed largely by those who study isolated rat α-cells (Gromada et al. 2007) and is debated largely by those who study α-cells in intact, primarily mouse islets and favor direct α-cell signaling of glucagon secretion by glucose (MacDonald et al. 2007). Given the evidence that both indirect and direct signaling occurs (Gromada et al. 2007; MacDonald et al. 2007), the clinically relevant question is, "What is the predominant signaling mechanism in humans?" Although that question remains to be answered unequivocally, there is increasing support for an important, albeit not exclusive, role of β-cell signaling in the regulation of α-cell glucagon secretion.

Systematic studies of glucagon secretion from isolated rat α-cells (Olsen et al. 2005; Gromada et al. 2007), along with translational studies of glucagon secretion in humans (Raju and Cryer 2005; Banarer et al. 2003; Gosmanov et al. 2005; Israelian et al. 2005; Cooperberg and Cryer, 2008), have led to renewed interest in the intra-islet insulin hypothesis. The cellular mechanisms of glucagon release from isolated rat α-cells are remarkably similar to those of insulin release from β-cells (Olsen et al. 2005; Gromada et al. 2007). Among the many parallels, low glucose concentrations decrease both insulin release from β-cells and glucagon release from isolated α-cells. That is in sharp contrast to the α-cell response to hypoglycemia in vivo (and to the response from isolated intact islets): low glucose levels decrease insulin secretion but increase glucagon secretion (Figure 3.7). The intra-islet insulin hypothesis (in vivo within intact islets, a decrease in β-cell secretion signals an increase in α-cell secretion in the setting of hypoglycemia) reconciles that apparent contradiction (Figure 3.7).

Whereas additional β-cell secretory products might well be involved in the intra-islet signaling of the glucagon response to hypoglycemia (Gromada et al. 2007; Zhou, Zhang et al. 2007), the fact that perfusion of the pancreas with an antibody to insulin causes glucagon release from the perfused pancreas (Maruyama et al. 1984) indicates that a decrease in intra-islet insulin is an important signal to glucagon secretion (and that the mechanism is, at least in part, endocrine rather than paracrine).

The intra-islet insulin hypothesis does not include a role for somatostatin, secreted from islet δ-cells, in the physiology or pathophysiology of glucagon secretion. If hypoglycemia decreases somatostatin secretion (Ipp et al. 1977), it is conceivable that a decrease in intra-islet somatostatin, as well as insulin, could normally signal increased glucagon secretion and that loss of that signal could explain loss of the glucagon response. However, selective destruction of β-cells, as in type 1 diabetes, results in loss of the glucagon response to hypoglycemia (Gerich et al. 1973), a finding that implicates a decrease in intra-islet insulin as the relevant signal to glucagon secretion.

There is now a body of evidence that the intra-islet insulin hypothesis for the regulation of glucagon secretion during hypoglycemia is operative in humans (Raju and Cryer 2005; Banarer et al. 2002; Gosmanov et al. 2005; Israelian et al. 2005; Cooperberg and Cryer 2008). First, intra-islet hyperinsuline-mia prevents the glucagon response to hypoglycemia in non-diabetic humans (Banarer et al. 2002). Second, reduction of the decrement in intra-islet insulin during the induction of hypo-glycemia decreases the glucagon response to hypoglycemia in humans (Raju and Cryer 2005; Gosmanov et al. 2005). Third, enhancement of the decrement in intra-islet insulin during the induction of hypoglycemia increases the glucagon response to hypoglycemia in humans (Israelian et al. 2005). Fourth, indirect, β-cell-mediated signaling also predominates over direct α-cell signaling during euglycemia and hyperglycemia in humans (Cooperberg and Cryer 2008). Thus, because a decrease in intra-islet insulin, in concert with a low plasma glucose concentration, normally signals an increase in glucagon secretion, loss of the intra-islet insulin signal plausibly explains loss of the glucagon response to hypoglycemia in insulin-deficient diabetes (Cryer 2004, 2008; Raju and Cryer 2005).

## Attenuated sympathoadrenal responses

The mechanism(s) of the key component of HAAF in diabetes, the attenuated central nervous system (CNS)–mediated sympathoadrenal response to falling plasma glucose concentrations, is not known. That causes hypoglycemia unawareness and, in the setting of absent decrements in insulin and absent increments in glucagon, causes defective glucose counterregu-lation, and thus HAAF and iatrogenic hypoglycemia in type 1 diabetes and advanced type 2 diabetes (Cryer 2004, 2008;

Dagogo-Jack et al. 1993; Segel et al. 2002). Clearly, however, it is different from that of loss of the insulin and glucagon responses to hypoglycemia, since the latter occur at the level of the diseased pancreatic islets, whereas the attenuated sympathoadrenal response involves the CNS (Figure 3.6).

Theoretically, the alteration that causes the glycemic thresholds for the sympathoadrenal and symptomatic (among other) responses to shift to lower plasma glucose concentrations after recent antecedent hypoglycemia (or after exercise and during sleep) could be in the CNS or in the afferent or efferent components of the sympathoadrenal system. Indeed, the finding of a reduced plasma metanephrine response to hypoglycemia in patients with type 1 diabetes and HAAF suggests a reduced adrenomedullary capacity to secrete epinephrine (de Galan et al. 2004). However, the finding that recurrent hypoglycemia reduces neuronal activation in the hypothalamus and in the intermediolateral cell column of the spinal cord in rats (Zhou, Fan et al. 2007) suggests that the alteration lies within the CNS. Potential CNS mechanisms include *1*) the systemic mediator hypothesis, *2*) the brain fuel transport hypothesis, and *3*) the brain metabolism hypothesis (Cryer 2005).

The systemic mediator hypothesis posits that increased circulating cortisol levels (or perhaps those of another systemic factor) during recent antecedent hypoglycemia (or exercise) act on the brain to reduce the sympathoadrenal (among other) responses to a given level of subsequent hypoglycemia (Davis et al. 1996, 1997a). Substantial antecedent cortisol elevations, produced by cortisol infusion or ACTH administration, do reduce the sympathoadrenal and symptomatic responses to subsequent hypoglycemia (Davis et al. 1996; McGregor et al. 2002). However, that appears to be an effect of supraphysiological cortisol concentrations. Less marked plasma cortisol elevations, to levels comparable to those that occur during hypoglycemia, do not reduce adrenomedullary or symptomatic responses to subsequent hypoglycemia (Raju et al. 2003; Goldberg et al. 2006). Furthermore, inhibition of the cortisol response to antecedent hypoglycemia (with metyrapone) does not prevent the effect of antecedent hypoglycemia to reduce the sympathoadrenal (or other) responses to subsequent hypoglycemia (Goldberg et al. 2006). There is also evidence that antecedent plasma epinephrine elevations do not cause HAAF (de Galan et al. 2003).

The brain fuel transport hypothesis posits that recent antecedent hypoglycemia causes increased blood-to-brain transport of glucose (or of an alternative metabolic fuel) and thus reduces sympathoadrenal (and other) responses to subsequent hypoglycemia (Boyle et al. 1994, 1995). However, global blood-to-brain glucose transport, measured with [1-$^{11}$C]glucose and positron emission tomography (PET), is not reduced in people with poorly controlled type 1 diabetes (Fanelli et al. 1998) and is not increased after recent antecedent hypoglycemia in non-diabetic individuals, a model of HAAF (Segel et al. 2001). Furthermore, global blood-to-brain [$^{11}$C]3-0-methylglucose (Bingham et al. 2002) and [$^{18}$F]deoxyglucose (Cranston et al. 2001; Dunn et al. 2007) transport, measured with PET, is not increased in type 1 diabetic patients with hypoglycemia unawareness. These data do not exclude increased regional blood-to-brain glucose transport, but the hypothesis was based on evidence of increased global brain glucose uptake (Boyle et al. 1994, 1995). Furthermore, in rodents, recent antecedent hypoglycemia does not increase regional extracellular glucose concentrations—measured by microdialysis in ventromedial hypothalamus (de Vries et al. 2003), brain stem (McCrimmon et al. 2003b), or hippocampus (McNay and Sherwin 2004)—during subsequent hypoglycemia. Theoretically, increased glucose flux into the brain could be coupled to increased brain glucose metabolism, and thus no change in the brain extracellular fluid glucose concentration, in the latter experiments (de Vries et al. 2003; McCrimmon et al. 2003b; McNay and Sherwin 2004). However, it is difficult to envision increased glucose transport into the brain as the signal that reduces the sympathoadrenal response to hypoglycemia in the absence of a higher brain extracellular fluid glucose concentration.

The finding of increased blood-to-brain acetate transport in people with diabetes (Mason et al. 2006) raises the possibility that increased monocarboxylate (e.g., lactate) transport into the brain might be a mechanism of HAAF. However, increased blood-to-brain lactate transport in type 1 diabetes and greater lactate transport in patients with HAAF remain to be demonstrated.

The brain metabolism hypothesis posits that some alteration in brain metabolism induced by recent antecedent hypoglycemia (and by prior exercise or by sleep) causes HAAF. The specific causative alteration remains to be identified. Because the hypothalamus can be seen as the central integrator of the sympathoadrenal response to hypoglycemia, much of the neuroscience research into the possible mechanisms of HAAF has been focused on that region of the brain (Cryer 2005, 2006). Alterations in the functions of glucose-excited and glucose-inhibited hypothalamic neurons induced by recent antecedent hypoglycemia, and therefore potentially involved in the pathogenesis of HAAF, include increased glucokinase activity (Levin et al. 2008), decreased AMP kinase activation (McCrimmon et al. 2008), decreased ATP-sensitive K$^+$ (K$_{ATP}$) channel activity (McCrimmon et al. 2005), increased urocortin III release (McCrimmon et al. 2006), increased γ-aminobutyric acid (GABA) release (Chan et al. 2007), and decreased brain insulin signaling (Fisher et al. 2005) among others. However, a coherent picture of the molecular and cellular alterations in hypothalamic function that lead to HAAF is only beginning to emerge (McCrimmon 2008; Sherwin 2008).

Whereas the primary alteration leading to HAAF could reside in the hypothalamus, the observed changes in hypothalamic function could be secondary to those in other brain regions. For example, the brain glycogen supercompensation hypothesis posits that the normally rather small brain astrocytic glycogen pool (Chapter 2) increases substantially after hypoglycemia and that expanded source of fuel within the brain results in a reduced sympathoadrenal response during subsequent hypoglycemia (Gruetter 2003). However, the evidence in rats that brain glycogen concentrations increase substantially above baseline after hypoglycemia (Choi et al. 2003) has been disputed (Herzog et al. 2008). It is perhaps relevant that approximately twofold post-hypoglycemic brain glycogen supercompensation was observed when hypoglycemia was terminated by glucose infusion resulting in substantial hyperglycemia (Choi et al. 2003) but not when hypoglycemia was terminated by free access to food (Herzog et al. 2008).

The mechanism of HAAF may well involve modulation of hypothalamic activity by an ultimately inhibitory cerebral network (Teves et al. 2004; Arbelaez et al. 2008). Measurements of regional cerebral blood flow with [$^{15}$O]water and positron emission tomography (PET) in humans indicate that hypoglycemia causes both *1*) a small (6–8%) generalized decrease in brain synaptic activity with a sharp decrease (25%) in the hippocampus and *2*) an increase in synaptic activity in a discrete system of interconnected brain regions including the medial prefrontal cortex, the lateral orbitofrontal cortex, the thalamus, the globus pallidus, and the peri-aqueductal grey (Teves et al. 2004). Recent antecedent hypoglycemia both reduces the sympathoadrenal and symptomatic responses to subsequent hypoglycemia, producing a model of HAAF in nondiabetic individuals, and causes a greater increase in synaptic activity in the dorsal midline thalamus in response to subsequent hypoglycemia (Arbelaez et al. 2008) (Figure 3.8). Because that brain region includes the paraventricular nucleus of the thalamus, which is known to mediate habituation of the hypothalamic-pituitary-adrenocortical response to recurrent restraint stress in rats (Jaferi and Bhatnagar 2006), it has been suggested that, in humans, increased dorsal midline thalamic activation might suppress the hypothalamic glucose sensor–initiated sympathoadrenal response to hypoglycemia, the key feature of HAAF in diabetes (Teves et al. 2004) (Figure 3.8).

Cranston et al. (Bingham et al. 2005) found a greater decrease in [18F]deoxyglucose uptake in the subthalamic region of the brain, centered in the hypothalamus, during hypoglycemia in patients with type 1 diabetes and hypoglycemia unawareness. That finding is consistent with the suggestion of increased thalamic inhibition of hypothalamic activity in HAAF (Arbelaez et al. 2008).

Given the neuroanatomical and functional connections of the dorsal midline thalamus, there may be a cerebral network (including medial prefrontal cortex, orbital prefrontal cortex, hippocampus, amygdala, and periaqueductal grey) that modulates dorsal midline thalamic inhibition of the sympathoadrenal

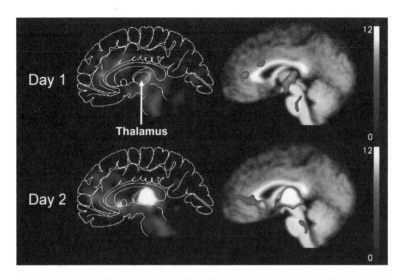

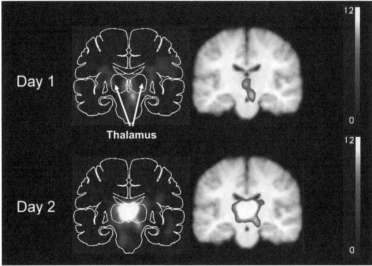

**Figure 3.8.** Increased dorsal midline thalamus synaptic activation, measured with $^{15}$O water and positron emission tomography, in a model of HAAF in nondiabetic humans. Reproduced from Arbelaez et al. 2008, with permission from the American Diabetes Association.

response to hypoglycemia (Arbelaez et al. 2008). If so, signaling of that network leading to increased dorsal midline thalamic inhibition of hypothalamic activity could lead to the reduced sympathoadrenal response to hypoglycemia that characterizes HAAF (Figure 3.6). The description of an array of differences in the patterns of [$^{18}$F]deoxyglucose uptake during hypoglycemia—in orbitofrontal cortex, amygdala, stratum, and brain stem, among other sites in patients with type 1 diabetes with and without unawareness (Cranston et al. 2001; Dunn et al. 2007)—is consistent with the participation of such a cerebral network in the pathogenesis of HAAF in diabetes.

## SUMMARY

Insulin excess of sufficient magnitude can cause iatrogenic hypoglycemia. However, in the vast majority of instances, it is the integrity of physiological and behavioral defenses against falling plasma glucose concentrations that determines whether an episode of relative, or even absolute, therapeutic hyperinsulinemia results in an episode of hypoglycemia. Thus, hypoglycemia is typically the result of the interplay of therapeutic insulin excess and compromised glycemic defenses (i.e., HAAF) in type 1 diabetes and advanced type 2 diabetes. The common denominator of the two components of HAAF—defective glucose counterregulation and hypoglycemia unawareness—is an attenuated sympathoadrenal response to a given level of hypoglycemia. In addition to therapeutic hyperinsulinemia, absent decrements in insulin and absent increments in glucagon, both the result of β-cell failure in type 1 diabetes and advanced type 2 diabetes, are prerequisites for defective glucose counterregulation. In that setting, attenuated epinephrine responses cause that clinical syndrome. Attenuated sympathoadrenal responses, largely reduced sympathetic neural responses, also cause the clinical syndrome of hypoglycemia unawareness. The attenuated sympathoadrenal responses, the key feature of HAAF, can be caused by recent antecedent hypoglycemia and prior exercise or sleep, perhaps among other causes. The fact that loss of the insulin and glucagon responses stems from β-cell failure explains why HAAF develops early in the course of type 1 diabetes but only later in the course of type 2 diabetes. That in turn explains why iatrogenic hypoglycemia becomes limiting to glycemic control early in type 1 diabetes but later in type 2 diabetes.

Understanding of this pathophysiology of glucose counterregulation in diabetes leads directly to insight into the risk factors for (Chapter 4), the definition and classification of (Chapter 5), and the prevention or treatment of (Chapter 6) clinical iatrogenic hypoglycemia in diabetes.

# Chapter 4.
# The Risk Factors for
# Hypoglycemia in Diabetes

The risk factors for hypoglycemia in people with diabetes (Cryer et al. 2003; Cryer 2004, 2008) (Table 4.1) follow directly from the pathophysiology of glucose counterregulation in diabetes (Chapter 3). The principle is that iatrogenic hypoglycemia in type 1 diabetes and advanced type 2 diabetes is typically the result of the interplay of relative or absolute therapeutic insulin excess and compromised physiological and behavioral defenses against falling plasma glucose concentrations, i.e., hypoglycemia-associated autonomic failure (HAAF) in diabetes.

## RELATIVE OR ABSOLUTE INSULIN EXCESS

The conventional risk factors for hypoglycemia in diabetes (Cryer et al. 2003; Cryer 2004, 2008) are based on the premise that relative or absolute therapeutic insulin excess is the sole determinant of risk. That may be either endogenous (secretagogue stimulated) or exogenous insulin excess. People with type 2 diabetes using an insulin secretagogue and people with type 1 diabetes or type 2 diabetes using insulin are at ongoing risk for episodes of hyperinsulinemia because of the pharmacokinetic imperfections of those therapies. Indeed, therapeutic hyperinsulinemia is a prerequisite for the development of hypoglycemia in diabetes (Chapter 3). Whereas those episodes can include absolute hyperinsulinemia, the conventional risk factors also focus on relative hyperinsulinemia, i.e., insulin levels insufficient to cause hypoglycemia under most conditions but high enough to cause hypoglycemia in the setting of decreased exogenous glucose delivery or endogenous glucose production, increased glucose utilization, or increased sensitivity to insulin, as well as decreased clearance of insulin (Table 4.1).

Absolute or relative therapeutic insulin excess occurs when insulin secretagogue or insulin doses are excessive, ill-timed, or of the wrong type. Relative insulin excess occurs under a variety

**Table 4.1.** Risk Factors for Hypoglycemia in Diabetes

**Relative or absolute insulin excess:**

1. Insulin or insulin secretagogue doses are excessive, ill-timed, or of the wrong type

2. Exogenous glucose delivery is decreased (e.g., after missed meals and during the overnight fast)

3. Endogenous glucose production is decreased (e.g., after alcohol ingestion)

4. Glucose utilization is increased (e.g., during and shortly after exercise)

5. Sensitivity to insulin is increased (e.g., after weight loss or improved glycemic control and in the middle of the night)

6. Insulin clearance is decreased (e.g., with renal failure)

**Hypoglycemia-associated autonomic failure:**

1. Absolute endogenous insulin deficiency

2. A history of severe hypoglycemia, hypoglycemia unawareness, or both as well as recent antecedent hypoglycemia, prior exercise, and sleep

3. Aggressive glycemic therapy per se (lower A1C levels, lower glycemic goals, or both)

of conditions. It occurs when exogenous glucose delivery is decreased, as it is after missed (or low-carbohydrate) meals and during the overnight fast; when endogenous glucose production is decreased, as it is after alcohol ingestion; when glucose utilization is increased, as it is during or shortly after exercise; and when sensitivity to insulin is increased, in the long term after weight loss or improved glycemic control and in the short term in the middle of the night. Insulin clearance is decreased with renal failure.

These are the risk factors people with diabetes and their caregivers deal with whenever hypoglycemia becomes a problem. Clearly, in a given patient, each of these needs to be considered carefully and the regimen adjusted appropriately. Nonetheless, these risk factors explain only a minority of episodes of hypoglycemia (DCCT 1991). In most instances, other risk factors, specifically those indicative of HAAF, determine whether a given episode of therapeutic hyperinsulinemia does, or does not, result in an episode of hypoglycemia (Chapter 3).

## HYPOGLYCEMIA-ASSOCIATED AUTONOMIC FAILURE

The risk factors for hypoglycemia indicative of HAAF (Cryer et al. 2003; Cryer 2004, 2008) (Table 4.1) include the degree of absolute endogenous insulin deficiency (Fukuda et al. 1998; DCCT 1997; Mühlhauser et al. 1997; Allen et al. 2001; Steffes et al. 2003; UK Hypo Group 2007); a history of severe hypoglycemia, hypoglycemia unawareness, or both (DCCT 1997; Mühlhauser et al. 1997; Allen et al. 2001; Wright et al. 2006); and conditions known to cause HAAF (recent antecedent hypoglycemia, prior exercise, or sleep) and aggressive glycemic therapy per se (DCCT 1997; Mühlhauser et al. 1997; Allen et al. 2001; Steffes et al. 2003; Wright et al. 2006; Lüddeke et al. 2007).

As discussed earlier, defective glucose counterregulation, one of the components of HAAF, develops in the setting of absent decrements in insulin and absent increments in glucagon, and both of these pathophysiological features stem fundamentally from β-cell failure (Chapter 3). Thus, the degree of absolute endogenous insulin deficiency determines both the extent to which insulin levels will not decrease and the extent to which glucagon levels will not increase as plasma glucose concentrations fall in response to therapeutic hyperinsulinemia. Longer duration of diabetes (and increasing age) are associated with loss of endogenous insulin secretion, early in type 1 diabetes and later in type 2 diabetes.

A history of severe hypoglycemia indicates, and a history of hypoglycemia unawareness implies, recent antecedent hypoglycemia. As discussed earlier (Chapter 3), recent antecedent hypoglycemia causes an attenuated sympathoadrenal response to subsequent hypoglycemia, the key feature of defective glucose counterregulation and the cause of hypoglycemia unawareness, which are the two components of HAAF, and thus the pathogenesis of iatrogenic hypoglycemia. In addition to recent antecedent hypoglycemia, prior exercise and sleep cause HAAF.

As documented in clinical trials with sample sizes large enough to demonstrate beneficial effects in type 1 diabetes (DCCT 1993; Reichard and Pihl 1994) and type 2 diabetes (Wright et al. 2006; ADVANCE 2008), and confirmed in a meta-analysis that included 12 smaller trials in type 1 diabetes (Egger et al. 1997), if all other factors are the same, patients treated to lower, compared with higher, A1C levels are at higher risk for hypoglycemia. Stated differently, studies with a control group treated to a higher A1C level consistently report higher rates of hypoglycemia in the group treated to a lower A1C level in type 1 diabetes (DCCT 1993; Reichard and Pihl 1994; Egger et al. 1997) and type 2 diabetes (Wright et al. 2006; ADVANCE 2008; ACCORD 2008). Indeed, lower mean plasma glucose concentrations and greater plasma glucose variability are also associated with a higher risk of hypoglycemia (Kilpatrick et al. 2007). That does not, of course, mean that one cannot both improve glycemic control and minimize the risk for hypoglycemia in individual patients (Cryer et al. 2003; Cryer 2004, 2008; Rossetti et al. 2008) (Chapter 6).

Improved glycemic control before and during pregnancy is particularly important in the short term because it improves pregnancy outcomes in women with type 1 diabetes. But, it increases the frequency of hypoglycemia substantially (Evers et al. 2002; Nielsen et al. 2008). In one series, 45% of 108 women with type 1 diabetes suffered severe hypoglycemia during their pregnancies; compared with a prepregnancy rate of 110 per 100 patient-years, the incidence was the equivalent of 530, 240, and 50 episodes per 100 patient-years in the first, second, and third trimesters, respectively (Neilsen et al. 2008). The risk factors for HAAF—previous severe hypoglycemia (Evers et al. 2002; Nielsen et al. 2008), impaired awareness of hypoglycemia (Nielsen et al. 2008), and lower A1C levels (Evers et al. 2002)—are also associated with higher rates of severe hypoglycemia in pregnant women with type 1 diabetes.

Finally, an association between an insertion/deletion polymorphism resulting in higher serum ACE activity and severe hypoglycemia, but not other hypoglycemias, has been reported in people with type 1 diabetes (Pedersen-Bjergaard et al. 2001, 2003; Nordfeldt and Samuelsson 2003). However, that polymorphism was not found to be associated with impaired awareness of hypoglycemia in type 1 diabetes (Holstein et al. 2006), was only weakly associated with severe hypoglycemia in a series of adults with type 1 diabetes (Zammitt et al. 2007), was not associated with severe hypoglycemia in children and adolescents with type 1 diabetes (Bulsara et al. 2007), and was not significantly associated with severe hypoglycemia in type 2 diabetes (Freathy et al. 2006).

# Chapter 5.
# The Clinical Definition and Classification of Hypoglycemia in Diabetes

## THE ALERT VALUE

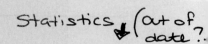 Statistics (out of date?..

The American Diabetes Association (ADA) Workgroup on Hypoglycemia (2005) defined hypoglycemia in diabetes as "all episodes of abnormally low plasma glucose concentration that expose the individual to potential harm." The workgroup recommended that people with drug-treated diabetes (implicitly those treated with an insulin secretagogue or insulin) become concerned about developing hypoglycemia at a plasma glucose concentration of ≤70 mg/dl (≤3.9 mmol/l) (ADA Workgroup on Hypoglycemia 2005). Within the error of self–plasma glucose monitoring (or continuous glucose-sensing) devices, that glucose level approximates the lower limit of the nondiabetic postabsorptive plasma glucose concentration range (Cryer 2001) and the normal glycemic thresholds for activation of physiological glucose counterregulatory systems (Cryer 2001) (Chapter 2), and is low enough to reduce glycemic defenses against subsequent hypoglycemia (Davis et al. 1997b), in nondiabetic individuals. That glucose level is higher than the plasma glucose levels required to produce neurogenic and neuroglycopenic symptoms (~54 mg/dl, 3.0 mmol/l) or to impair brain function in nondiabetic individuals (Cryer 2001, 2007) and substantially higher than the glucose levels that do so in people with well-controlled diabetes (Cryer 2007; Amiel et al.

1988), although people with poorly controlled diabetes sometimes have symptoms at somewhat higher glucose levels (Amiel et al. 1988; Boyle et al. 1988).

Use of a 70 mg/dl (3.9 mmol/l) plasma glucose alert level generally gives the patient time to take action to prevent a clinical hypoglycemic episode. Also, in practice, self–plasma glucose monitoring is usually done with devices that are not precise analytical instruments, particularly at low glucose levels (Diabetes Research in Children Network Study Group 2003). The recommended alert level provides some margin for their inaccuracy.

The recommended generic alert level does not mean that people with diabetes should always treat at an estimated plasma glucose concentration of ≤70 mg/dl. Rather, it indicates that they should consider an action ranging from repeating the measurement in the short term through behavioral changes such as avoiding exercise or driving to carbohydrate ingestion and subsequent regimen adjustments.

The plasma glucose alert value of ≤70 mg/dl (≤3.9 mmol/l) has been criticized as being too high because glucose levels are occasionally lower than that in nondiabetic individuals and its use would lead to an overestimation of the frequency of clinically important hypoglycemia (Amiel et al. 2008). The former is true, albeit generally during prolonged fasting. The latter is wide of the mark. The issue is not to estimate the frequency of clinically important hypoglycemia. It is to prevent clinically important hypoglycemia. Notably, after criticizing the ADA recommended alert value, the authors recommended a lower limit of the therapeutic plasma glucose concentration of 72–81 mg/dl (4.0–4.5 mmol/l) (Amiel et al. 2008).

## CLASSIFICATION OF HYPOGLYCEMIA

The ADA Workgroup also recommended a classification of hypoglycemia in diabetes (ADA Workgroup on Hypoglycemia 2005) (Table 5.1). That includes severe hypoglycemia, using a definition that has been used widely since the initial report of the Diabetes Control and Complications Trial (DCCT 1993), documented symptomatic hypoglycemia and asymptomatic hypoglycemia, as well as probable symptomatic hypoglycemia and relative hypoglycemia. The latter category reflects the fact that patients with poorly controlled diabetes can experience

**Table 5.1.** American Diabetes Association Workgroup on Hypoglycemia Classification of Hypoglycemia in People with Diabetes

**Severe hypoglycemia.** An event requiring assistance of another person to actively administer carbohydrate, glucagon, or other resuscitative actions. Plasma glucose measurements may not be available during such an event, but neurological recovery attributable to the restoration of plasma glucose to normal is considered sufficient evidence that the event was induced by a low plasma glucose concentration.

**Documented symptomatic hypoglycemia.** An event during which typical symptoms of hypoglycemia are accompanied by a measured plasma glucose concentration ≤70 mg/dl (≤3.9 mmol/l).

**Asymptomatic hypoglycemia.** An event not accompanied by typical symptoms of hypoglycemia but with a measured plasma glucose concentration ≤70 mg/dl (≤3.9 mmol/l).

**Probable symptomatic hypoglycemia.** An event during which symptoms typical of hypoglycemia are not accompanied by a plasma glucose determination but that was presumably caused by a plasma glucose concentration ≤70 mg/dl (≤3.9 mmol/l).

**Relative hypoglycemia.** An event during which the person with diabetes reports any of the typical symptoms of hypoglycemia and interprets those as indicative of hypoglycemia, with a measured plasma glucose concentration >70 mg/dl (>3.9 mmol/l) but approaching that level.

symptoms of hypoglycemia as their plasma glucose concentrations fall into the physiological range (Amiel et al. 1988; Boyle et al. 1988).

## QUANTITATION OF HYPOGLYCEMIA UNAWARENESS

Hypoglycemia unawareness, or impaired awareness of hypoglycemia (IAH) since there is a spectrum from normal awareness through reduced awareness to complete unawareness (Frier and Fisher 1999), is a component of HAAF (Chapter 3) and a risk factor for iatrogenic hypoglycemia (Chapter 4). Three methods have been used to attempt to systematically identify affected patients. The method of Gold et al. (1994) asks the patient to complete a seven-point scale ranging from 1, always aware, to 7, never aware in response to the question, "Do you know when your hypos are commencing?" A score of ≥4 is considered to indicate IAH. The method of Clarke et al. (1995) asks eight questions about the patient's hypoglycemia experience. A score of ≥4 is considered to indicate IAH. The method of Pedersen-Bjergaard et al. (2001) asks the patient to select one of the terms "always," "usually," "sometimes," or "never" in response to the question, "Can you feel when you are low?" Any response other than always is considered to indicate IAH. In a comparison of the three methods in 80 patients with type 1 diabetes, Geddes et al. (2007) found prevalences of IAH of 24, 26, and 62%, respectively, with the three methods. Over the subsequent 4 weeks, patients classified as having IAH by the Gold and Clarke methods had higher rates of low self-monitored plasma glucose concentrations and lower neurogenic symptom scores during hypoglycemia (<54 mg/dl, <3.0 mmol/l). They also had

22- and 32-fold higher incidences and 10- and 11-fold higher prevalences of severe hypoglycemia, respectively. Those classified as having IAH by the Pedersen-Bjergaard method did not have significantly higher rates of low self-monitored plasma glucose concentrations or lower neurogenic symptom scores during hypoglycemia, although the trends were in those directions. They did have a higher incidence and prevalence of severe hypoglycemia. In response, Pedersen-Bjergaard et al. (2007) indicated that with their more recent version, which is based on the question, "Do you have symptoms when you have a hypo?", the answer "always" implies normal awareness, "usually" impaired awareness, and "occasionally" or "never" severely impaired awareness (unawareness). With that, they find unawareness in 10–15% of patients but impaired awareness in 40–50% (Pedersen-Bjergaard et al. 2007).

## QUANTITATION OF ENDOGENOUS INSULIN DEFICIENCY

Normally, insulin secretion adapts to maintain plasma glucose concentrations within, or return them to, the postabsorptive physiological range. Insulin is secreted from pancreatic β-cells into the hepatic portal venous circulation, and ~50% is cleared by the liver. C-peptide, the peptide cleaved from proinsulin to yield insulin, is secreted in equimolar quantities with insulin. But C-peptide is not cleared by the liver. Therefore, plasma C-peptide concentrations provide an index of endogenous insulin secretion. Indeed, plasma C-peptide data can be used to calculate rates of insulin secretion (Eaton et al. 1980; Polonsky et al. 1986; Heller and Cryer 1991a).

Plasma C-peptide concentrations are ~0.5–1.5 ng/ml (~0.2–

0.5 nmol/l) after an overnight fast in healthy euglycemic individuals. Normally, the concentrations decrease as plasma glucose levels decline within the physiological range and become
virtually indistinguishable from zero if glucose levels fall below
the physiological range (Heller and Cryer 1991a).

Absolute insulin deficiency is a fundamental feature of
defective glucose counterregulation and thus HAAF (Chapter
3) and is a risk factor for iatrogenic hypoglycemia (Chapter 4).
One approach to the quantitation of endogenous insulin deficiency is to define the plasma C-peptide concentrations that
identify patients with clinical type 1 diabetes, since, after the
"honeymoon" period, they have virtually complete endogenous insulin deficiency from a metabolic perspective. In general, fasting plasma C-peptide concentrations ≤0.6 ng/ml
(≤0.2 nmol/l) characterize type 1 diabetes (DCCT 1986; Gjessing et al. 1989; Service et al. 1997), although a higher cutoff
value has been reported (Berger et al. 2000) (Table 5.2). A
wider range of glucagon-stimulated plasma C-peptide levels

**Table 5.2.** Fasting, Stimulated (6 Minutes after 1.0 mg of Glucagon
Intravenously), and Random Plasma C-peptide Concentrations in
Patients Judged Clinically to Have Type 1 Diabetes

|  | Fasting | Stimulated | Random |
|---|---|---|---|
| DCCT 1986 | ≤0.6 ng/ml | ≤1.5 ng/ml | — |
|  | ≤0.2 nmol/l | ≤0.5 nmol/l | — |
| Gjessing et al. 1989 | <0.6 ng/ml | <1.0 ng/ml | — |
|  | <0.2 nmol/l | <0.3 nmol/l | — |
| Service et al. 1997 | <0.5 ng/ml | ↑<0.2 ng/ml | — |
|  | <0.2 nmol/l | ↑<0.1 nmol/l | — |
| Berger et al. 2000 | ≤1.2 ng/ml | ≤1.8 ng/ml | ≤1.5 ng/ml |
|  | ≤0.4 nmol/l | ≤0.6 nmol/l | ≤0.5 nmol/l |

has been reported to identify type 1 diabetes (DCCT 1986; Gjessing et al. 1989; Service et al. 1997; Berger et al. 2000) (Table 5.2). Residual β-cell function continues for a longer period of time in adults compared with adolescents with type 1 diabetes (DCCT 1987).

Interestingly, among the 262 patients judged clinically to have type 2 diabetes by Service and colleagues (Service et al. 1997), 20 (8%) displayed an insulin-deficient plasma C-peptide pattern initially, and an additional 33 (13%) did so on at least one occasion during subsequent testing. Unfortunately, the proportion of those patients who had late-onset autoimmune diabetes (i.e., type 1 diabetes), as opposed to progression of type 2 diabetes to absolute endogenous insulin deficiency, is not known.

# Chapter 6.
# The Prevention and Treatment of Hypoglycemia in Diabetes

## PREVENTION OF HYPOGLYCEMIA: HYPOGLYCEMIA RISK FACTOR REDUCTION

It is, of course, preferable to prevent, rather than to treat, hypoglycemia in people with diabetes. The prevention of hypoglycemia requires the practice of hypoglycemia risk factor reduction (Cryer et al. 2003; Cryer 2008). That involves four steps: *1)* Acknowledge the problem. *2)* Apply the principles of aggressive glycemic therapy (Cryer et al. 2003; Cryer 2008; Bolli 2003; Davis and Alonso 2004; de Galan et al. 2006; Boyle and Zrebiec 2007; Rossetti et al. 2008). *3)* Consider the conventional risk factors (Chapter 4) (Table 4.1). *4)* Consider the risk factors indicative of hypoglycemia-associated autonomic failure (HAAF) in diabetes (Chapter 4) (Table 4.1).

### Acknowledge the problem

The issue of hypoglycemia should be addressed in every patient contact, or at least with those with insulin secretagogue or insulin-treated diabetes. Patient concerns about the reality, or even the possibility, of hypoglycemia can be a barrier to glycemic control (Gonder-Frederick et al. 2006; Nordfeldt and Ludvigsson 2005). Indeed, some studies suggest that people with insulin-treated diabetes are more concerned about the possibility of an episode of hypoglycemia than about the long-term complications of diabetes (Nordfeldt and Ludvigsson 2005). Yet, patients are often reluctant to volunteer their concerns. They should be given the explicit opportunity to do so. It is also often helpful to question close associates of the patient, since they may have observed clues to episodes of hypoglycemia not recognized by the patient. Even if no concerns are expressed, examination of the self–plasma glucose monitoring record (or continuous glucose-sensing data) may disclose that hypoglycemia is a problem.

## Apply the principles of aggressive glycemic therapy

If hypoglycemia is a problem, each of the principles of aggressive glycemic therapy (Cryer et al. 2003; Cryer 2008; Bolli 2003; Davis and Alonso 2004; de Galan et al. 2006; Boyle and Zrebiec 2007; Rossetti et al. 2008) (Table 6.1) should be considered and applied.

Patient education and empowerment are fundamentally important. As the therapeutic regimen becomes progressively more complex—early in type 1 diabetes and later in type 2 diabetes—the success of glycemic management becomes progressively more dependent on the many management decisions and the skills of the well-informed person with diabetes. Without

**Table 6.1.** Principles of Aggressive Glycemic Therapy of Diabetes

| | |
|---|---|
| 1. | Patient education and empowerment |
| 2. | Frequent self–plasma glucose monitoring (and in some instances continuous glucose sensing) |
| 3. | Flexible and appropriate insulin (and other drug) regimens |
| 4. | Individualized glycemic goals |
| 5. | Ongoing professional guidance and support |

those, it will often not be successful.

In addition to basic training about diabetes, people with insulin secretagogue or insulin-treated diabetes need to be taught about the anticipation, recognition, and treatment of hypoglycemia (Cox et al. 2004). They need to know how their medications can cause hypoglycemia. They need to know the common symptoms of hypoglycemia and, over time, to learn their individual most meaningful symptoms. They need to know how to treat (and not over-treat) hypoglycemia. Close associates, such as spouses, need to be taught how to recognize an episode of severe hypoglycemia and how to administer parenteral glucagon. Patients need to understand the conventional risk factors for hypoglycemia (Table 4.1), including the effects of the dose and timing of their individual secretagogue or insulin preparation(s) as well as the effects of missed meals and the overnight fast, alcohol, and exercise. They also need to know that episodes of hypoglycemia (a risk factor for HAAF [Table 4.1]) signal an increased likelihood of future, often more severe, episodes. Indeed, Cox and colleagues have shown that increasingly frequent low self-monitored glucose levels identify increasing risk of imminent severe hypoglycemia (Kovatchev et al. 1998, 2003; Cox et al. 2007). In a systematic analysis of prospectively obtained self–plasma glucose monitoring data and of the occurrence of severe hypoglycemia, they found that a recent increase in their calculated low blood glucose index detected ~60% of imminent (within 24 hours) episodes of severe hypoglycemia in both type 1 diabetes and insulin-treated type 2 diabetes (Cox et al. 2007). Finally, patients using a continuous glucose sensor need to learn how to apply those data to their attempts to minimize hypoglycemia as well as hyperglycemia. Again, the successful glycemic management of type 1 diabetes and of advanced type 2 diabetes is critically dependent on a well-informed person with diabetes.

It is reasonable to anticipate that frequent self–plasma glucose monitoring (supplemented in some instances by continuous glucose sensing) will provide insight leading to rational modifications of the therapeutic regimen, although additional critical evidence on that point is needed. Logically, that would become more key to short-term management decisions as the regimen becomes more complex. Ideally, patients should monitor their plasma glucose level whenever they suspect hypoglycemia. That would not only confirm or deny hypoglycemia; it would also help the person learn the key symptoms of their hypoglycemic episodes and might lead to regimen adjustments. It is particularly important for people with hypoglycemia unawareness to monitor their plasma glucose level before performing a critical task such as driving.

Self–plasma glucose monitoring provides a glucose estimate at only one point in time and therefore does not indicate whether glucose levels are rising, stable, or falling toward hypoglycemia. That limitation is being addressed by the development of technologies for continuous glucose sensing. Those technologies are evolving (Hovorka 2005; Ellis et al. 2007; Deiss et al. 2006; Wilson et al. 2007; Buckingham et al. 2007). Hopefully, they will ultimately lead to closed-loop insulin replacement (Steil et al. 2006).

Among the commonly used sulfonylureas, glyburide [glibenclamide] is most often associated with hypoglycemia (Holstein and Egberts 2003; Gangji et al. 2007). The use of long-acting basal insulin analogs (e.g., glargine, detemir) in a multiple daily injection (MDI) insulin regimen reduces at least the incidence of nocturnal hypoglycemia, perhaps that of total, symptomatic, and nocturnal hypoglycemia in type 1 diabetes and type 2 diabetes (Hirsch 2005; Horvath et al. 2007; Gough 2007). The use of a rapid-acting prandial insulin analog (e.g., lispro, aspart, glulisine) reduces the incidence of nocturnal hypoglycemia at least in type 1 diabetes (Hirsch 2005; Gough 2007). Although it is conceptually attractive, the superiority of continuous subcutaneous insulin infusion (CSII) with an analog over MDI with analogs with respect to the frequency and severity of hypoglycemia at comparable levels of glycemic control remains to be established convincingly.

A systematic review of 15 randomized controlled trials (13 in type 1 diabetes) comparing CSII and MDI, published since 2002, disclosed nonsignificant trends favoring CSII for severe, nocturnal, and minor hypoglycemia (Fatourechi et al. In press). Elevated end-of-study A1C levels (mean 7.7%) were the rule, five studies excluded patients with a history of severe hypoglycemia or hypoglycemia unawareness, and eight studies used NPH insulin as the basal insulin in the MDI regimen (Fatourechi et al. In press). Thus, the relative safety of CSII over MDI with a long-acting insulin analog as the basal insulin (and a rapid-acting analog as the prandial insulin), particularly in patients with tight glycemic control, hypoglycemia unawareness, or both, remains to be documented convincingly. A positive view is that CSII results in slightly lower A1C levels without increasing the risk of hypoglycemia (Fatourechi et al. In press; Jeitler et al. 2008). However, the shortcomings of many of the trials remain, including the frequent failure to treat to recommended glycemic goals, to compare CSII with contemporary MDI regimens using insulin analogs, and to focus on patients at particularly high risk of hypoglycemia. A systematic review of six randomized controlled trials in pregnant women with diabetes did not show a significant advantage of CSII over MDI (Mukho-padhyay et al. 2007).

In addition to the use of insulin analogs (Hirsch 2005; Horvath et al. 2007; Gough 2007), approaches to the prevention of nocturnal hypoglycemia include attempts to produce sustained delivery of exogenous carbohydrate or sustained endogenous glucose production throughout the night (Raju et al. 2006). With respect to the former approach, a conventional bedtime snack or bedtime administration of uncooked cornstarch has not been found to be effective (Raju et al. 2006). With respect to the latter approach, bedtime administration of the epinephrine-simulating $\beta_2$-adrenergic agonist terbutaline has been shown to prevent nocturnal hypoglycemia in patients with aggressively treated type 1 diabetes in preliminary studies (Raju et al. 2006), but it also caused hyperglycemia the following morning. This promising off label use of terbutaline warrants a sufficiently powered, placebo-controlled, randomized trial.

In people with diabetes, the generic glycemic goal is an A1C level as close to the nondiabetic range as can be accomplished safely in a given patient (ADA 2008; Qaseem et al. 2007) at a given point in the evolution of his or her diabetes. Nonetheless, there is substantial long-term benefit from reducing A1C from higher to lower, although still above desirable, levels (DCCT 1993; UKPDS 1998a, 1998b; Lachin et al. 2008). Therefore, glycemic goals should be individualized.

Finally, because the glycemic management of diabetes is empirical, caregivers should work with the individual patient over time to find the best method of glycemic control at a given time in the course of that patient's diabetes. Care is best accomplished by a team that includes, in addition to a physician, professionals trained in, and dedicated to, translating the standards of care (ADA 2008) into care of individual patients and making full use of modern communication and computing technologies.

## Consider the conventional risk factors

In a patient with iatrogenic hypoglycemia, each of the conventional risk factors, those that result in relative or absolute insulin excess (Table 4.1), should be considered carefully, and the therapeutic regimen should be adjusted appropriately. In addition to the dose, type, and timing of insulin or insulin secretagogue medications, those risk factors include conditions in which exogenous glucose delivery or endogenous glucose production is decreased, glucose utilization or sensitivity to insulin is increased, or insulin clearance is reduced.

## Consider the risk factors indicative of HAAF

Risk factors indicative of HAAF include the degree of absolute endogenous insulin deficiency, a history of severe hypoglycemia, hypoglycemia unawareness, or both as well as any relationship between hypoglycemic episodes and recent antecedent hypoglycemia, prior exercise or sleep, and lower A1C levels (Table 4.1). Unless the cause is easily remediable, a history of severe hypoglycemia should prompt consideration of a fundamental regimen adjustment. Without that, the risk of a subsequent episode of severe hypoglycemia is high (Kovatchev et al. 1998, 2003; Cox et al. 2007; DCCT 1997). Given a history of hypoglycemia unawareness, a 2- to 3-week period of scrupulous avoidance of hypoglycemia, which may require acceptance of somewhat higher glycemic goals in the short term, is advisable, since that can be expected to restore awareness (Fanelli et al. 1993, 1994b; Cranston et al. 1994; Dagogo-Jack et al. 1994). A history of late post-exercise hypoglycemia, nocturnal hypoglycemia, or both should prompt appropriately timed regimen adjustments (generically, less insulin action, more carbohydrate ingestion, or both) or, failing these, a pharmacological treatment (Raju et al. 2006).

To date, the only established approach to reversal of hypoglycemia unawareness, and at least in part the attenuated epinephrine component of defective glucose counterregulation, is a period of scrupulous avoidance of hypoglycemia (Fanelli et al. 1993, 1994b; Cranston et al. 1994; Dagogo-Jack et al. 1994). Reversal of the attenuated sympathoadrenal response would correct the key feature of HAAF and therefore reduce the risk of hypoglycemia. In that regard, the finding that administration of the selective serotonin reuptake inhibitor (SSRI) sertraline increased the sympathoadrenal response to hypoglycemia (including the reduced response that followed recurrent hypoglycemia) in rats (Sanders et al. 2008) and that of the SSRI fluoxetine increased the plasma epinephrine and muscle sympathetic nerve activity responses (but not the symptomatic or glucagon responses) to hypoglycemia in patients with type 1 diabetes (Briscoe et al. 2008a, 2008b) is of interest.

## TREATMENT OF HYPOGLYCEMIA

Hypoglycemia causes functional brain failure that is corrected after the plasma glucose concentration is raised in the vast majority of instances (Cryer 2007). Profound, prolonged hypoglycemia can cause brain death (Cryer 2007). The former is presumably the result of transient brain fuel deprivation, but the latter is not. Neuronal death is thought to be caused by a series of mechanisms including massive release of the excitatory neurotransmitter glutamate (Cryer 2007; Suh et al. 2007).

Clearly, the plasma glucose concentration should be raised to normal levels promptly. Data from a rodent model of extreme hypoglycemia suggest that post-treatment glycemia contributes to neuronal death (Suh et al. 2007). Although the clinical extrapolation of that finding is unclear (Cryer 2007), it may be that post-hypoglycemia hyperglycemia should be avoided, at least after an episode of profound, prolonged hypoglycemia.

In people with diabetes, most episodes of asymptomatic hypoglycemia (detected by self–plasma glucose monitoring or glucose sensing) or of mild-moderate symptomatic hypoglycemia are effectively self-treated by ingestion of glucose tablets or carbohydrate-containing juice, soft drinks, candy, other snacks, or a meal (Cryer 2008; MacCuish 1993; Wiethop and Cryer 1993a). A reasonable dose is 20 g glucose (Cryer 2008; Wiethop and Cryer 1993a) (Figure 6.1). Clinical improve-

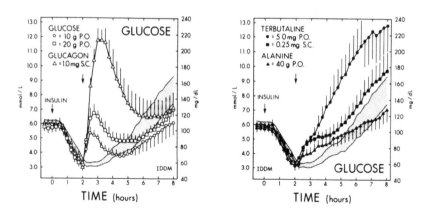

**Figure 6.1.** Mean (+SE) plasma glucose concentrations during insulin-induced hypoglycemia in patients with type 1 diabetes (IDDM) in the absence of an intervention (shaded area) and after the indicated interventions. S.C., subcutaneous, P.O., per os. From Wiethop and Cryer 1993b, reproduced with permission of the American Diabetes Association.

ment should occur in 15–20 minutes. However, in the setting of ongoing hyperinsulinemia, the glycemic response to oral glucose is transient—typically <2 hours (Wiethop and Cryer 1993a). Thus, ingestion of a more substantial snack or meal shortly after the plasma glucose level is raised is generally advisable.

Parenteral treatment is required when a hypoglycemic patient is unwilling (because of neuroglycopenia) or unable to take carbohydrate orally. Glucagon, injected subcutaneously or intramuscularly in a usual dose of 1.0 mg in adults by an associate of the patient, is often used in people with diabetes. That can be lifesaving, but it often causes substantial, albeit transient, hyperglycemia (Figure 6.1), and it can cause nausea or even vomiting. Smaller doses of glucagon (e.g., 150 µg), repeated if necessary, have been found to be effective without side effects in children (Haymond and Schreiner 2001). Because it stimulates insulin secretion, glucagon might be less useful in patients other than those with type 1 diabetes or advanced type 2 diabetes. Indeed, glucagon has been reported to cause hypoglycemia in nondiabetic individuals (Cryer et al. In press). Because it acts primarily by stimulating hepatic glycogenolysis, glucagon treatment is ineffective in glycogen-depleted individuals (e.g., after a binge of alcohol ingestion).

Although glucagon can be administered intravenously by medical personnel, in that setting, intravenous glucose is the standard parenteral therapy. A common initial dose of intravenous glucose is 25 g (Cryer 2008; MacCuish 1993); lower doses could be used in a setting in which plasma glucose concentrations can be measured serially. The glycemic response to intravenous glucose is of course transient in the setting of ongoing hyperinsulinemia. A subsequent glucose infusion is often

## Table 6.2. Clinical Practice Guidelines (Cryer et al. In press)

1.  We suggest that individuals with diabetes become concerned about the possibility of developing hypoglycemia when the self-monitored blood glucose concentration is falling rapidly or is ≤70 mg/dl (≤3.9 mmol/l).

2.  Given the established long-term microvascular, and potential macrovascular, benefits of glycemic control, we recommend that the therapeutic glycemic goal be the lowest mean glycemia (e.g., A1C) that can be accomplished safely in a given patient at a given point in the progression of that individual patient's diabetes.

3.  We recommend that the prevention of hypoglycemia in diabetes involves addressing the issue in each patient contact and, if hypoglycemia is a problem, making adjustments in the regimen based on review and application of the principles of aggressive glycemic therapy—patient education and empowerment, frequent self–blood glucose monitoring, flexible and appropriate insulin or insulin secretagogue regimens, individualized glycemic goals, and ongoing professional guidance and support—and consideration of each of the known risk factors for hypoglycemia.

4.  We recommend that both the conventional risk factors and those indicative of compromised defenses against hypoglycemia be considered in a patient with recurrent treatment-induced hypoglycemia. The conventional risk factors are excessive or ill-timed dosing of, or wrong type of, insulin or insulin secretagogue and conditions under which exogenous glucose delivery or endogenous glucose production is decreased, glucose utilization is increased, sensitivity to insulin is increased, or insulin clearance is decreased. Compromised defenses against hypoglycemia are indicated by the degree of endogenous insulin deficiency, a history of severe hypoglycemia, hypoglycemia unawareness, or both, as well as recent antecedent hypoglycemia, prior exercise or sleep, and lower glycemic goals per se.

5.  With a history of hypoglycemia unawareness (i.e., recurrent hypoglycemia without symptoms), we recommend a 2- to 3-week period of scrupulous avoidance of hypoglycemia, with the anticipation that awareness of hypoglycemia will return in many patients.

6.  Unless the cause is easily remediable, we recommend that an episode of severe hypoglycemia should lead to a fundamental review of the treatment regimen.

7.  We recommend that urgent treatment of hypoglycemia should be accomplished by ingestion of carbohydrates if that is feasible and by parenteral glucagon or glucose if the former is not feasible.

needed, and food should be provided orally as soon as the patient is able to ingest it safely.

The duration of a hypoglycemic episode is a function of its cause. An episode caused by a rapid-acting insulin secretagogue or insulin analog will be relatively brief, and that caused by a long-acting insulin analog will be substantially longer. A sulfonylurea overdose, or that of a long-acting insulin analog, can result in prolonged hypoglycemia requiring hospitalization.

## CLINICAL PRACTICE GUIDELINES

Many of the principles discussed in this book were incorporated, by a panel organized by The Endocrine Society, into a set of clinical practice guidelines for the evaluation and management of adult hypoglycemic disorders (Cryer et al. In press). The development of the guidelines included an assessment of the strength of the supporting evidence, resulting in suggestions based on weaker evidence and recommendations based on stronger evidence. The suggestions and recommendations concerning hypoglycemia in people with diabetes are listed in Table 6.2.

# Chapter 7.
# Perspective on Hypoglycemia in Diabetes

iabetes is an increasingly common chronic disease. Its
human and economic costs are large and, despite
advances in therapy, are growing because of the
increasing prevalence of diabetes. Since the introduction of
insulin therapy in 1922, it has been possible to prevent early
death from diabetic ketoacidosis or hyperosmolar coma and to
eliminate symptoms of uncontrolled hyperglycemia in the vast
majority of patients. However, by the mid-20th century it was
apparent that the early insulin therapies did not prevent the
long-term microvascular and macrovascular complications of
diabetes. Diabetes became the leading cause of end-stage renal
disease requiring dialysis or transplantation, of blindness with its
onset in working-age adults, and of nontraumatic amputations,
and most people with diabetes died from cardiovascular disease.
There were important practical advances in diabetes care in the
late 20th century. Those included the development of A1C measurements to quantitate overall glycemic control, self–plasma
glucose monitoring (and more recently, continuous glucose
sensing) to assess short-term glycemic control, insulin analogs
with more favorable (albeit less than ideal) pharmacokinetic
profiles, an array of new drugs that lower plasma glucose concentrations early in the course of type 2 diabetes, and the concept of a diabetes care team, among others. Since the landmark
Diabetes Control and Complications Trial in type 1 diabetes,

published in 1993, many studies, including the U.K. Prospective Diabetes Study in type 2 diabetes, have led to widespread consensus that long-term glycemic control prevents or delays at least the microvascular complications of diabetes. Nonetheless, those complications are still a reality for many people with diabetes. Furthermore, the impact of the barrier of iatrogenic hypoglycemia, the limiting factor in the glycemic management of many people with diabetes, has been more widely appreciated (Chapter 1).

Glycemic control, which is the focus of this book because its topic is hypoglycemia in diabetes, is but one aspect of the management of diabetes. For example, it is now clear that blood lipid and blood pressure control, as well as blood glucose control, are fundamentally important to the prevention or delay of the vascular complications of diabetes. However, while it is now possible to drive LDL cholesterol to subphysiological levels and to normalize blood pressure pharmacologically, usually without major side effects, in most people with diabetes, it is still not possible to maintain euglycemia over a lifetime of diabetes in the vast majority of patients because of the barrier of iatrogenic hypoglycemia.

Based on insight into the physiology of glucose counterregulation (Chapter 2) and its pathophysiology, and the relationship of the latter to clinical hypoglycemia, in diabetes (Chapter 3), many risk factors for iatrogenic hypoglycemia have been identified (Chapter 4) and a working definition and classification of hypoglycemia in diabetes has been proposed (Chapter 5). Thus, it is now possible to both improve glycemic control and reduce the risk of hypoglycemia in many people with diabetes (Chapter 6).

It is important for both diabetes caregivers and people with diabetes to keep the problem of iatrogenic hypoglycemia in perspective. The underlying principle of the glycemic management of diabetes is that maintenance of glycemia as close to the nondiabetic range as can be accomplished safely over time is in the patient's best interests. It reduces the development of microvascular complications and may reduce that of macrovascular complications. The extent to which that goal can be met is a function of many factors, including the type of diabetes and the stage in the evolution of diabetes in an individual patient. Type 2 diabetes is, by far, the more common type of diabetes. Early in the course of type 2 diabetes, hyperglycemia may respond to lifestyle changes, specifically weight loss, or to plasma glucose–lowering drugs that do not raise circulating insulin levels and therefore should not, and probably do not, cause hypoglycemia. Those include the biguanide metformin, thiazolidinediones, and α-glucosidase inhibitors that do not cause hyperinsulinemia. They also include GLP-1 receptor agonists and dipeptidyl peptidase-IV (DPP-IV) inhibitors, which raise insulin levels only in the presence of hyperglycemia. In theory, when such drugs are effective, there is no reason not to accelerate their dosing until euglycemia is achieved in the absence of nonglycemic side effects. The reality, however, is that either initially, or over time, as patients with type 2 diabetes become progressively more insulin deficient, these drugs (even in combination) fail to provide glycemic control. Insulin secretagogues, a sulfonylurea or a glinide, are also effective early in the course of type 2 diabetes, although these raise endogenous insulin levels and therefore introduce the possibility of iatrogenic hypoglycemia. Nonetheless, as emphasized in Chapter 1, the frequency of iatrogenic hypoglycemia is relatively low (at least with current glycemic goals) during treatment with an insulin secretagogue, or even with insulin, early in the course of type 2 diabetes when glucose counterregulatory defenses are intact. Thus, over most of the course of the most common type of diabetes, it is possible to achieve a meaningful degree of glycemic control with no risk or relatively low risk of iatrogenic hypoglycemia. Clearly, that is beneficial to those patients. Therefore, it is fundamentally important that concerns about the risk of hypoglycemia should not be used as an excuse for poor glycemic control by diabetes caregivers or by people with diabetes in most instances. Rather, both should strive to achieve and maintain the greatest glycemic control that can be accomplished safely in a given patient with diabetes at a given stage of his or her diabetes.

All people with type 1 diabetes, and ultimately most with type 2 diabetes, require treatment with insulin. Insulin is demonstrably effective. Given in sufficient doses, it will lower plasma glucose concentrations in all people with diabetes. Insulin therapy is life-saving in type 1 diabetes and is necessary in those with advanced (i.e., absolutely insulin-deficient) type 2 diabetes. In the latter patients, it should be introduced earlier, rather than later, when other therapies fail to achieve glycemic control. The difficulty of course is that, while it is demonstrably effective, insulin is not demonstrably safe. Because of the pharmacokinetic imperfections of insulin therapy, particularly in the setting of compromised glucose counterregulation (the syndromes of defective glucose counterregulation and hypoglycemia unawareness and therefore hypoglycemia-associated autonomic failure) that develop early in type 1 diabetes and later in type 2 diabetes, it is limited by the barrier of iatrogenic hypoglycemia. Therefore, the goal of long-term euglycemia is not feasible in such patients with current insulin regimens.

Although it can be minimized in many patients, the problem

of iatrogenic hypoglycemia in type 1 diabetes and advanced type 2 diabetes has not been solved. Diabetes will someday be cured and prevented, but no one knows when that will be accomplished. Short of that, elimination of hypoglycemia from the lives of people with diabetes will likely be accomplished by the development of methods that provide plasma glucose–regulated insulin replacement (i.e., closed-loop insulin therapy) or secretion (i.e., implantation of insulin-secreting cells). In the meantime, innovative research, ranging from studies of the fundamental molecular and cellular mechanisms of the physiology and pathophysiology of glucose counterregulation to clinical trials of novel approaches to the prevention of iatrogenic hypoglycemia, is clearly needed if we are to improve the lives of all people affected by diabetes by eliminating hypoglycemia.

# Bibliography

Abraira C, Colwell JA, Nuttall FQ, Swain CT, Nagel NJ, Comstock JP, Emanuele NV, Levin SR, Henderson W, Lee HS. 1995. Veterans Affairs Cooperative Study on Glycemic Control and Complications in Type II Diabetes (VA CSCM). *Diabetes Care* 18:1113–1123.

Action to Control Cardiovascular Risk in Diabetes Study Group [ACCORD]. 2008. Effects of intensive glucose lowering in type 2 diabetes. *N Engl J Med* 358:2545–2559.

Adler GK, Bonyhay I, Failing H, Waring E, Dotson S, Freeman R. In press. Antecedent hypoglycemia impairs cardiovascular function—implications for rigorous glycemic control. *Diabetes.*

ADVANCE Collaborative Group [ADVANCE]. 2008. Intensive blood glucose control and vascular outcomes in patients with type 2 diabetes. *N Engl J Med* 358:2560–2572.

Akram K, Pedersen-Bjergaard U, Carstensen B, Borch-Johnsen K, Thorsteinsson B. 2006. Frequency and risk factors for severe hypoglycaemia in insulin-treated type 2 diabetes: a cross sectional survey. *Diabet Med* 23:750–756.

Allen C, LeCaire T, Palta M, Daniels K, Meredith M, D'Alessio DJ, for the Wisconsin Diabetes Registry Project. 2001. Risk factors for frequent and severe hypoglycemia in type 1 diabetes. *Diabetes Care* 24:1878–1881.

American Diabetes Association [ADA]. 2008. Standards of medical care in diabetes: 2008. *Diabetes Care* 31 (Suppl. 1):S5–S54.

American Diabetes Association Workgroup on Hypoglycemia. 2005. Defining and reporting hypoglycemia in diabetes. *Diabetes Care* 28:1245–1249.

Amiel SA, Dixon T, Mann R, Jameson K. 2008. Hypoglycaemia in type 2 diabetes. *Diabet Med* 25:245–254.

Amiel SA, Sherwin RS, Simonson DC, Tamborlane WV. 1988. Effect of intensive insulin therapy on glycemic thresholds for counterregulatory hormone release. *Diabetes* 37:901–907.

Amos AF, McCarty DJ, Zimmet P. 1997. The rising global burden of diabetes and its complications: estimates and projections to the year 2010. *Diabet Med* 14 (Suppl 5):S1–S85.

Arbelaez AM, Powers WJ, Videen TO, Price JL, Cryer PE. 2008. Attenuation of counterregulatory responses to recurrent hypoglycemia by active thalamic inhibition: a mechanism for hypoglycemia-associated autonomic failure. *Diabetes* 57:470–475.

Banarer S, Cryer PE. 2003. Sleep-related hypoglycemia-associated autonomic failure in type 1 diabetes: reduced awakening from sleep during hypoglycemia. *Diabetes* 52:1195–1203.

Banarer S, McGregor VP, Cryer PE. 2002. Intraislet hyperinsulinemia prevents the glucagon response to hypoglycemia despite an intact autonomic response. *Diabetes* 51:958–965.

Benedict C, Hallschmid M, Hatke A, Schultes B, Fehm HL, Born J, Kern W. 2004. Intranasal insulin improves memory in humans. *Psychoneuroendocrinology* 29:1326–1334.

Benedict C, Hallschmid M, Schultes B, Born J. 2007. Intranasal insulin to improve memory function in humans. *Neuroendocrinology* 86:136–142.

Benedict L, Nelson CA, Schunk E, Sullwold K, Seaquist ER. 2006. Effect of insulin on the brain activity obtained during visual and memory tasks in healthy human subjects. *Neuroendocrinology* 83:20–26.

Berger B, Stenström G, Sundkvist G. 2000. Random C-peptide in the classification of diabetes. *Scand J Clin Lab Invest* 60:687–694.

Bergman RN. 2007. Orchestration of glucose homeostasis. *Diabetes* 56:1489–1501.

Berk MA, Clutter WE, Skor D, Shah SD, Gingerich RP, Parvin CA, Cryer PE. 1985. Enhanced glycemic responsiveness to epinephrine in insulin-dependent diabetes mellitus is the result of the inability to secrete insulin. *J Clin Invest* 75:1842-1851.

Berlin I, Grimaldi A, Payan C, Sachon C, Bosquet F, Thervet F, Puech AJ. 1987. Hypoglycemic symptoms and decreased β-adrenergic sensitivity in insulin dependent diabetic patients. *Diabetes Care* 10:742–747.

Bingham EM, Dunn JT, Smith D, Sutcliffe-Goulden J, Reed LJ, Marsden PK, Amiel SA. 2005. Differential changes in brain glucose metabolism during hypoglycaemia accompany loss of hypoglycaemia awareness in men with type 1 diabetes mellitus: an [¹¹C]-3-O-methyl-D-glucose PET study. *Diabetologia* 48:2080–2089.

Bingham EM, Hopkins D, Smith D, Pernet A, Hallet W, Reed L, Marsden PK, Amiel SA. 2002. The role of insulin in human brain glucose metabolism: an ¹⁸fluoro-deoxyglucose positron emission tomography study. *Diabetes* 51:3384–3390.

Bliss M. 1992. *Banting: A Biography.* 2nd ed. Toronto, University of Toronto Press, pp. 74–75.

Bolen S, Feldman L, Vassy J, Wilson L, Yeh H-C, Marinopoulos S, Wiley C, Selvin E, Wilson R, Bass EB, Brancati FL. 2007. Systematic review: comparative effectiveness and safety of oral mediations for type 2 diabetes mellitus. *Ann Intern Med* 147:386–399.

Bolli GB. 2003. Treatment and prevention of hypoglycemia and its unawareness in type 1 diabetes mellitus. *Rev Endocr Metab Dis* 4:335–341.

Bolli G, De Feo P, Compagnucci P, Cartechini MG, Angeletti F, Santeusanio F, Brunetti P, Gerich JE. 1983. Abnormal glucose counterregulation in insulin dependent diabetes: interaction of anti-insulin antibodies and impaired glucagon and epinephrine secretion. *Diabetes* 32:134–141.

Bolli GB, De Feo P, De Cosmo S, Perriello G, Ventura MM, Massi-Benedetti M, Santeusanio F, Gerich JE, Brunetti P. 1984. A reliable and reproducible test for adequate glucose counter-regulation in type 1 diabetes mellitus. *Diabetes* 33:732–737.

Bolli G, De Feo P, Perriello G, De Cosmo S, Ventura M, Campbell P, Brunetti P, Gerich JE. 1985. Role of hepatic autoregulation in defense against hypoglycemia in humans. *J Clin Invest* 75:1623–1631.

Bottini P, Boschetti E, Pampanelli S, Ciofetta M, Del Sindaco P, Scionti L, Brunetti P, Bolli GB. 1997. Contribution of autonomic neuropathy to reduced plasma adrenaline responses to hypoglycemia in IDDM: evidence for a non-selective defect. *Diabetes* 46:814–823.

Boyle PJ, Cryer PE. 1991. Growth hormone, cortisol, or both are involved in defense against, but are not critical to recovery from, hypoglycemia. *Am J Physiol Endocrinol Metab* 260:E395–E402.

Boyle PJ, Kempers SF, O'Connor AM, Nagy RJ. 1995. Brain glucose uptake and unawareness of hypoglycemia in patients with insulin dependent diabetes mellitus. *N Engl J Med* 333:1726–1731.

Boyle PJ, Nagy RJ, O'Connor AM, Kempers SF, Yeo RA, Qualls C. 1994. Adaptation in brain glucose uptake following recurrent hypoglycemia. *Proc Natl Acad Sci USA* 91:9352–9356.

Boyle PJ, Schwartz NS, Shah SD, Clutter WE, Cryer PE. 1988. Plasma glucose concentrations at the onset of hypoglycemic symptoms in patients with poorly controlled diabetes and in nondiabetics. *N Engl J Med* 318:1487–1492.

Boyle PJ, Shah SD, Cryer PE. 1989. Insulin, glucagon, and catecholamines in prevention of hypoglycemia during fasting in humans. *Am J Physiol Endocrinol Metab* 256:E651–E661.

Boyle PJ, Zrebiec J. 2007. Management of diabetes-related hypoglycemia. *Southern Med J* 100:183–194.

Breckenridge SM, Cooperberg BA, Arbelaez AM, Patterson BW, Cryer PE. 2007. Glucagon, in concert with insulin, supports the postabsorptive plasma glucose concentration in humans. *Diabetes* 56:2442–2448.

Briscoe VJ, Ertl AC, Tate DB, Blair HM, Davis SN. 2008a. Effects of the selective serotonin reuptake inhibitor, fluoxetine, on counterregulatory responses to hypoglycemia in individuals with T1DM. *Diabetes* 57:3315-3322.

Briscoe VJ, Ertl AC, Tate DB, Dawling S, Davis SN. 2008b. Effects of a selective serotonin reuptake inhibitor, fluoxetine, on counterregulatory responses to hypoglycemia in healthy individuals. *Diabetes* 57:2453–2460.

Bruce S, Tack C, Patel J, Pacak K, Goldstein DS. 2002. Local sympathetic function in human skeletal muscle and adipose tissue assessed by microdialysis. *Clin Auton Res* 12:13–19.

Brunkhorst FM, Engel C, Bloos F, et al. for the German Competence Network Sepsis (SepNet). 2008. Intensive insulin therapy and pentastarch resuscitation in severe sepsis. *N Engl J Med* 358:125–139.

Buckingham B, Caswell K, Wilson DM. 2007. Real-time continuous glucose monitoring. *Curr Opin Endocrinol Diabetes Obes* 14:288–295.

Bulsara MK, Holman CDJ, van Bockxmeer FM, Davis EA, Gallego PH, Beilby JP, Palmer LJ, Choong C, Jones TW. 2007. The relationship between ACE genotype and risk of severe hypoglycaemia in a large population-based cohort of children and adolescents with type 1 diabetes. *Diabetologia* 50:965–971.

Caprio S, Tamborlane WV, Zych K, Gerow K, Sherwin RS. 1993. Loss of potentiating effect of hypoglycemia on the glucagon response to hyperaminoacidemia in IDDM. *Diabetes* 42:550–555.

Chan O, Lawson M, Zhu W, Beverly JL, Sherwin RS. 2007. ATP-sensitive $K^+$ channels regulate the release of GABA in the ventromedial hypothalamus during hypoglycemia. *Diabetes* 56:1120–1126.

Cherrington AD. 2001. Control of glucose production in vivo by insulin and glucagon. In *Handbook of Physiology. Section 7, The Endocrine System. Volume II, The Endocrine Pancreas and Regulation of Metabolism.* Jefferson LS, Cherrington AD, Eds. New York, Oxford University Press, pp. 759–785.

Choi IY, Seaquist ER, Gruetter R. 2003. Effect of hypoglycemia on brain glycogen metabolism in vivo. *J Neurosci Res* 72:25–32.

Christensen NJ, Norsk P. 2005. The fallacy of plasma noradrenaline spillover measurements. *Acta Physiol Scand* 183:333–334.

Clarke DD, Sokoloff L. 1994. Circulation and energy metabolism of the brain. In *Basic Neurochemistry: Molecular, Cellular and Medical Aspects.* 5th ed. Siegel G, Agranoff B, Albers RW, Molinoff P, Eds. New York, Raven Press, pp. 645–680.

Clarke WL, Cox DJ, Gonder-Frederick LA, Julian D, Schlundt D, Polonsky W. 1995. Reduced awareness of hypoglycemia in IDDM adults: a prospective study of hypoglycemia frequency and associated symptoms. *Diabetes Care* 18:517–522.

Clarke WL, Santiago JV, Thomas L, Haymond MW, Ben-Galim E, Cryer PE. 1979. Adrenergic mechanisms in recovery from hypoglycemia in man: adrenergic blockade. *Am J Physiol Endocrinol Metab* 236:E147–E152.

Cooperberg BA, Cryer PE. 2008. The intraislet insulin hypothesis: type 1 diabetes as a model of isolated alpha-cell glucagon secretion (abstract). *Diabetes* 57:A7.

Cox DJ, Gonder-Frederick L, Ritterband L, Clarke W, Kovatchev BP. 2007. Prediction of severe hypoglycemia. *Diabetes Care* 30:1370-1373.

Cox DJ, Kovatchev B, Koev D, Koeva L, Dachev S, Tcharaktchiev D, Protopopova A, Gonder-Frederick L, Clarke W. 2004. Hypoglycemia anticipation, awareness and treatment training (HAATT) reduces occurrence of severe hypoglycemia among adults with type 1 diabetes mellitus. *Int J Behav Med* 11:212–218.

Craft S, Newcomer J, Kanne S, Dagogo-Jack S, Cryer P, Sheline Y, Luby J, Dagogo-Jack A, Alderson A. 1996.

Memory improvement following induced hyperinsuline-mia in Alzheimer's disease. *Neurobiol Aging* 17:123–130.

Cranston I, Lomas J, Maran A, Macdonald I, Amiel SA. 1994. Restoration of hypoglycaemia awareness in patients with long-duration insulin-dependent diabetes. *Lancet* 344:283–287.

Cranston I, Reed LJ, Marsden PK, Amiel SA. 2001. Changes in regional brain [18]F-fluorodeoxyglucose uptake at hypo-glycemia in type 1 diabetic men associated with hypoglyce-mia unawareness and counter-regulatory failure. *Diabetes* 50:2329–2336.

Cryer PE. 1981. Glucose counterregulation in man. *Diabetes* 30:261–264.

———. 1992. Iatrogenic hypoglycemia as a cause of hypogly-cemia-associated autonomic failure in IDDM: a vicious cycle. *Diabetes* 41:255–260.

———. 1993. Catecholamines, pheochromocytoma and dia-betes. *Diabetes Reviews* 1:309–317.

———. 1997. *Hypoglycemia: Pathophysiology, Diagnosis and Treatment*. New York, Oxford University Press, pp. 1–177.

———. 2001. The prevention and correction of hypoglyce-mia. In *Handbook of Physiology. Section 7, The Endocrine System. Volume II, The Endocrine Pancreas and Regulation of Metabolism*. Jefferson LS, Cherrington AD, Eds. New York, Oxford University Press, pp. 1057–1092.

———. 2004. Diverse causes of hypoglycemia-associated autonomic failure in diabetes. *N Engl J Med* 350:2272–2279.

———. 2005. Mechanisms of hypoglycemia-associated autonomic failure and its component syndromes in diabetes. *Diabetes* 54:3592–3601.

———. 2006a. Hypoglycaemia: the limiting factor in the glycaemic management of the critically ill? *Diabetologia* 49:1722–1725.

———. 2006b. Mechanisms of sympathoadrenal failure and hypoglycemia in diabetes. *J Clin Invest* 116:1470–1473.

———. 2007. Hypoglycemia, functional brain failure, and brain death. *J Clin Invest* 117:868–870.

———. 2008. Glucose homeostasis and hypoglycemia. In *Williams Textbook of Endocrinology*. 11th ed. Kronenberg H, Melmed S, Polonsky KS, Larsen PR, Eds. Philadelphia, Elsevier, pp. 1503–1533.

Cryer PE, Axelrod L, Grossman AB, Heller SR, Montori VM, Seaquist ER, Service FJ. In press. Evaluation and management of adult hypoglycemic disorders. *J Clin Endocrinol Metab*.

Cryer PE, Davis SN, Shamoon H. 2003. Hypoglycemia in diabetes. *Diabetes Care* 26:1902–1912.

Dagogo-Jack SE, Craft S, Cryer PE. 1993. Hypoglycemia-associated autonomic failure in insulin-dependent diabetes mellitus. *J Clin Invest* 91:819–828.

Dagogo-Jack S, Rattarasarn C, Cryer PE. 1994. Reversal of hypoglycemia unawareness, but not defective glucose counterregulation, in IDDM. *Diabetes* 43:1426–1434.

Davis S, Alonso MD. 2004. Hypoglycemia as a barrier to glycemic control. *J Diabetes Complications* 18:60–68.

Davis SN, Shavers C, Costa F, Mosqueda-Garcia R. 1996. Role of cortisol in the pathogenesis of deficient counterregulation after antecedent hypoglycemia in normal humans. *J Clin Invest* 98:680–691.

Davis SN, Shavers C, Davis B, Costa F. 1997a. Prevention of an increase in plasma cortisol during hypoglycemia preserves subsequent counterregulatory responses. *J Clin Invest* 100:429–438.

Davis SN, Shavers C, Mosqueda-Garcia R, Costa F. 1997b. Effects of differing antecedent hypoglycemia on subsequent counterregulation in normal humans. *Diabetes* 46:1328–1335.

Deckert T, Poulsen JE, Larsen M. 1978. Prognosis of diabetics with diabetes before the age of 31. I. Survival, cause of deaths and complications. *Diabetologia* 14:363–370.

De Feo P, Perriello G, De Cosmo S, Ventura MM, Campbell PJ, Brunetti P, Gerich JE, Bolli GB. 1986. Comparison of glucose counterregulation during short-term and prolonged hypoglycemia in normal humans. *Diabetes* 35:563–569.

De Feo P, Perriello G, Torlone E, Fanelli C, Ventura MM, Santeusanio F, Brunetti P, Gerich JE, Bolli GB. 1991a. Evidence against important catecholamine compensation for absent glucagon counterregulation. *Am J Physiol Endocrinol Metab* 260:E203–E212.

De Feo P, Perriello G, Torlone E, Fanelli C, Ventura MM, Santeusanio F, Brunetti P, Gerich JE, Bolli GB. 1991b. Contribution of adrenergic mechanisms to glucose counterregulation in humans. *Am J Physiol Endocrinol Metab* 261:E725–E736.

De Feo P, Perriello G, Torlone E, Ventura MM, Fanelli C, Santeusanio F, Brunetti P, Gerich JE, Bolli GB. 1989b. Contribution of cortisol to glucose counterregulation in humans. *Am J Physiol Endocrinol Metab* 257:E35–E42.

De Feo P, Perriello G, Torlone E, Ventura MM, Santeusanio F, Brunetti P, Gerich JE, Bolli GB. 1989a. Demonstration of a role for growth hormone in glucose counterregulation. *Am J Physiol Endocrinol Metab* 256:E835–E843.

de Galan BE, De Mol P, Wennekes L, Schouwenberg BJJ, Smits P. 2006. Preserved sensitivity to $\beta_2$-adrenergic receptor agonists in patients with type 1 diabetes mellitus and hypoglycemia unawareness. *J Clin Endocrinol Metab* 91:2878–2881.

de Galan BE, Rietjens SJ, Tack CJ, Van der Werf SP, Sweep CGJ, Lenders JWM, Smits P. 2003. Antecedent adrenaline attenuates the responsiveness to, but not the release of, counterregulatory hormones during subsequent hypoglycemia. *J Clin Endocrinol Metab* 88:5462–5467.

de Galan BE, Schouwenberg BJJW, Tack CJ, Smits P. 2006. Pathophysiology and management of recurrent hypoglycaemia and hypoglycaemia unawareness in diabetes. *Neth J Med* 64:269–279.

de Galan BE, Tack CJ, Willemsen JJ, Sweep CGJ, Smits P, Lenders JWM. 2004. Plasma metanephrine levels are decreased in type 1 diabetic patients with a severely impaired epinephrine response to hypoglycemia, indicating reduced stores of epinephrine. *J Clin Endocrinol Metab* 89:2057–2061.

de Heer J, Holst JJ. 2007. Sulfonylurea compounds uncouple the glucose dependence of the insulinotropic effect of glucagon-like peptide-1. *Diabetes* 56:438–443.

de Vries MG, Arseneau LM, Lawson ME, Beverly JL. 2003. Extracellular glucose in rat ventromedial hypothalamus during acute and recurrent hypoglycemia. *Diabetes* 52:2767–2773.

Deiss D, Hartmann R, Schmidt J, Kordonouri O. 2006. Results of a randomized controlled cross-over trial on the effect of continuous subcutaneous glucose monitoring (CGMS) on glycaemic control in children and adolescents with type 1 diabetes. *Exp Clin Endocrinol Diabetes* 114:63–67.

DeRosa MA, Cryer PE. 2004. Hypoglycemia and the sympathoadrenal system: neurogenic symptoms are largely the result of sympathetic neural, rather than adrenomedullary, activation. *Am J Physiol Endocrinol Metab* 287:E32–E41.

Diabetes Control and Complications Trial Research Group [DCCT]. 1986. The Diabetes Control and Complications Trial: design and methodologic considerations for the feasibility phase. *Diabetes* 35:530–545.

———. 1987. Effects of age, duration and treatment of insulin-dependent diabetes mellitus on residual β-cell function:

observations during eligibility testing for the Diabetes Control and Complications Trial (DCCT). *J Clin Endocrinol Metab* 65:30–36.

———. 1991. Epidemiology of severe hypoglycemia in the Diabetes Control and Complications Trial. *Am J Med* 90:450–459.

———. 1993. The effect of intensive treatment of diabetes on the development and progression of long-term complications in insulin dependent diabetes mellitus. *N Engl J Med* 329:977–986.

———. 1995. The relationship of glycemic exposure (HbA$_{1C}$) to the risk of development and progression of retinopathy in the Diabetes Control and Complications Trial. *Diabetes* 44:968–983.

———. 1996. Influence of intensive diabetes treatment on quality-of-life outcomes in the Diabetes Control and Complications Trial. *Diabetes Care* 19:195–203.

———. 1997. Hypoglycemia in the Diabetes Control and Complications Trial. *Diabetes* 46:271–286.

Diabetes Control and Complications Trial/Epidemiology of Diabetes Interventions and Complications Research Group. 2000. Retinopathy and nephropathy in patients with type 1 diabetes four years after a trial of intensive therapy. *N Engl J Med* 342:381–389.

———. 2005. Intensive diabetes treatment and cardiovascular disease in patients with type 1 diabetes. *N Engl J Med* 353:2643–2653.

———. 2007. Long-term effect of diabetes and its treatment on cognitive function. *N Engl J Med* 356:1842–1852.

Diabetes Research in Children Network (DirecNet) Study Group. 2003. A multicenter study of the accuracy of the One Touch Ultra home glucose meter in children with type 1 diabetes. *Diabetes Technology and Therapeutics* 5:933–941.

Diem P, Redmon JB, Abid M, Moran A, Sutherland DER, Halter JB, Robertson RP. 1990. Glucagon, catecholamine and pancreatic polypeptide secretion in type 1 diabetic recipients of pancreatic allografts. *J Clin Invest* 86:2008–2013.

Donnelly LA, Morris AD, Frier BM, Ellis JD, Donnan PT, Durrant R, Band MM, Reekie G, Leese GP, for the DARTS/MEMO Collaboration. 2005. Frequency and predictors of hypoglycaemia in type 1 and insulin-treated type 2 diabetes: a population-based study. *Diabet Med* 22:749–755.

Dunn JT, Cranston I, Marsden PK, Amiel SA, Reed LJ. 2007. Attenuation of amygdala and frontal cortical responses to low blood glucose concentration in asymptomatic hypoglycemia in type 1 diabetes. *Diabetes* 56:2766–2773.

Eaton RP, Allen RC, Schade DS, Erickson KM, Standefer J. 1980. Prehepatic insulin production in man: kinetic analysis using peripheral connecting peptide behavior. *J Clin Endocrinol Metab* 51:520–528.

Edgerton DS, Lautz M, Scott M, Everett CA, Stettler KM, Neal DW, Chu CA, Cherrington AD. 2006. Insulin's direct effects on the liver dominate the control of hepatic glucose production. *J Clin Invest* 116:521–527.

Egger M, Davey Smith G, Stettler C, Diem P. 1997. Risk of adverse effects of intensified treatment in insulin-dependent diabetes mellitus: a meta-analysis. *Diabet Med* 14:919–928.

Ellis SL, Bookout T, Garg SK, Izuora KE. 2007. Use of continuous glucose monitoring to improve diabetes mellitus management. *Endocrinol Metab Clinics N A* 36 (Suppl. 2):46–68.

Eisenhofer G. 2005. Sympathetic nerve function: assessment of radioisotope dilution analysis. *Clin Auton Res* 15:264–283.

Eisenhofer G, Kopin IJ, Goldstein DS. 2004. Catecholamine metabolism: a contemporary view with implications for physiology and medicine. *Pharmacological Reviews* 56:331–349.

Ertl AC, Davis SN. 2004. Evidence for a vicious cycle of exercise and hypoglycemia in type 1 diabetes mellitus. *Diabetes Metab Res Rev* 20:124–130.

Evers IM, ter Braak EWMT, de Valk HW, van der Schoot B, Janssen N, Visser GHA. 2002. Risk indicators predictive of severe hypoglycemia during the first trimester of type 1 diabetic pregnancy. *Diabetes Care* 25:554–559.

Fagius J. 2003. Sympathetic nerve activity in metabolic control: some basic concepts. *Acta Physiol Scand* 177:337–343.

Fanelli CG, De Feo P, Porcellati F, Perriello G, Torlone E, Santeusanio F, Brunetti P, Bolli GB. 1992. Adrenergic mechanisms contribute to the late phase of hypoglycemic glucose counterregulation in humans by stimulating lipolysis. *J Clin Invest* 89:2005–2013.

Fanelli CG, Dence CS, Markham J, Videen TO, Paramore DS, Cryer PE, Powers WJ. 1998. Blood-to-brain glucose transport and cerebral glucose metabolism are not reduced in poorly controlled type 1 diabetes. *Diabetes* 47:1444–1450.

Fanelli CG, Epifano L, Rambotti AM, Pampanelli S, Di Vincenzo A, Modarelli F, Lepore M, Annibale B, Ciofetta M, Bottini P, Porcellati F, Scionti L, Santeusanio F, Brunetti P, Bolli GB. 1993. Meticulous prevention of hypoglycemia normalizes the glycemic thresholds and magnitude of most of neuroendocrine responses to, symptoms of, and cognitive function during hypoglycemia in intensively treated patients with short-term IDDM. *Diabetes* 42:1683–1689.

Fanelli C, Pampanelli S, Epifano L, Rambotti AM, Ciofetta M, Modarelli F, Di Vincenzo A, Annibale B, Lepore M, Lalli C, Del Sindaco P, Brunetti P, Bolli GB. 1994a. Relative roles of insulin and hypoglycaemia on induction of neuroendocrine responses to, symptoms of, and deterioration of cognitive function in hypoglycaemia in male and female humans. *Diabetologia* 37:797–807.

Fanelli C, Pampanelli S, Epifano L, Rambotti AM, Di Vincenzo A, Modarelli F, Ciofetta M, Lepore M, Annibale B, Torlone E, Perriello G, De Feo P, Santeusanio F, Brunetti P, Bolli GB. 1994b. Long-term recovery from unawareness, deficient counterregulation and lack of cognitive dysfunction during hypoglycemia, following institution of rational, intensive therapy in IDDM. *Diabetologia* 37:1265–1276.

Fanelli CG, Paramore DS, Hershey T, Terkamp C, Ovalle F, Craft S, Cryer PE. 1998. Impact of nocturnal hypoglycemia on hypoglycemic cognitive dysfunction in type 1 diabetes. *Diabetes* 47:1920–1927.

Fatourechi MM, Kudva YC, Murad MH, Elamin MB, Tabini CC, Montori VM. In press. Hypoglycemia with intensive insulin therapy. A systematic review and meta-analysis of randomized trials of continuous subcutaneous insulin infusion versus multiple daily injections. *J Clin Endocrinol Metab*

Feltbower RG, Bodansky HJ, Patterson CC, Parslow RC, Stephenson CR, Reynolds C, McKinney PA. 2008. Acute complications and drug misuse are important causes of death for children and young adults with type 1 diabetes. *Diabetes Care* 31:922–926.

Fisher SJ, Brüning JC, Lannon S, Kahn CR. 2005. Insulin signaling in the central nervous system is critical for the normal sympathoadrenal response to hypoglycemia. *Diabetes* 54:1447–1451.

Freathy RM, Lonnen KF, Steele AM, Minton JAL, Frayling TM, Hattersley AT, MacLeod KM. 2006. The impact of the angiotensin-converting enzyme insertion/deletion polymorphism on severe hypoglycemia in type 2 diabetes. *Review of Diabetic Studies* 3:76–81.

Frier BM, Fisher BM. 1999. Impaired hypoglycemia awareness. In *Hypoglycaemia in Clinical Diabetes.* Fisher BM, Frier

BM, Eds. Chichester, U.K., John Wiley & Sons, pp. 111–146.

Fritsche A, Stefan N, Häring H, Gerich J, Stumvoll M. 2001. Avoidance of hypoglycemia restores hypoglycemia awareness by increasing β-adrenergic sensitivity in type 1 diabetes. *Ann Intern Med* 134:729–736.

Fukuda M, Tanaka A, Tahara Y, Ikegami H, Yamamoto Y, Kumahara Y, Shima K. 1988. Correlation between minimal secretory capacity of pancreatic β-cells and stability of diabetic control. *Diabetes* 37:81–88.

Galassetti P, Mann S, Tate D, Neill RA, Costa F, Wasserman DH, Davis SN. 2001. Effects of antecedent prolonged exercise on subsequent counterregulatory responses to hypoglycemia. *Am J Physiol Endocrinol Metab* 280:E908–E917.

Gangji AS, Cukierman T, Gerstein HC, Goldsmith GH, Clase CM. 2007. A systematic review and meta-analysis of hypoglycemia and cardiovascular events. *Diabetes Care* 30:389–394.

Garber AJ, Cryer PE, Santiago JV, Haymond MW, Pagliara AS, Kipnis DM. 1976. The role of adrenergic mechanisms in the substrate and hormonal response to insulin-induced hypoglycemia in man. *J Clin Invest* 58:7–15.

Geddes J, Schopman JE, Zammitt NN, Frier BM. 2008. Prevalence of impaired awareness of hypoglycaemia in adults with type 1 diabetes. *Diabet Med* 25:501–504.

Geddes J, Wright RJ, Zammitt NN, Deary IJ, Frier BM. 2007. An evaluation of methods of assessing impaired awareness of hypoglycemia in type 1 diabetes. *Diabetes Care* 30:1868–1870.

Gerich JE. 1988. Glucose counterregulation and its impact on diabetes mellitus. *Diabetes* 37:1608–1617.

———. 1989. Oral hypoglycemic agents. *N Engl J Med* 321:1231–1245.

Gerich J, Davis J, Lorenzi M, Rizza R, Bohannon N, Karam J, Lewis S, Kaplan R, Schultz T, Cryer P. 1979. Hormonal mechanisms of recovery from insulin-induced hypoglycemia in man. *Am J Physiol Endocrinol Metab* 236:E380–E385.

Gerich JE, Langlois M, Noacco C, Karam J, Forsham P. 1973. Lack of glucagon response to hypoglycemia in diabetes: evidence for an intrinsic pancreatic alpha-cell defect. *Science* 182:171–173.

Gjessing HJ, Matzen LE, Faber OK, Frølund A. 1989. Fasting plasma C-peptide, glucagon stimulated plasma C-peptide and urinary C-peptide in relation to clinical type of diabetes. *Diabetologia* 32:305–311.

Gold AE, MacLeod KM, Frier BM. 1994. Frequency of severe hypoglycemia in patients with type 1 diabetes and impaired awareness of hypoglycemia. *Diabetes Care* 17:697–703.

Goldberg PA, Weiss R, McCrimmon RJ, Hintz EV, Dziura J, Sherwin RS. 2006. Antecedent hypercortisolemia is not primarily responsible for generating hypoglycemia-associated autonomic failure. *Diabetes* 55:1121–1126.

Gonder-Frederick LA, Fisher CD, Ritterband LM, Cox DJ, Hou L, DasGupta AA, Clarke WL. 2006. Predictors of fear of hypoglycemia in adolescents with type 1 diabetes and their parents. *Pediatr Diabetes* 7:215–222.

Gosmanov NR, Szoke E, Israelian Z, Smith T, Cryer PE, Gerich JE, Meyer C. 2005. Role of the decrement in intraislet insulin for the glucagon response to hypoglycemia in humans. *Diabetes Care* 28:1124–1131.

Gough SCL. 2007. A review of human and analogue insulin trials. *Diabetes Res Clin Pract* 77:1–15.

Gromada J, Franklin I, Wollheim CB. 2007. Alpha cells of the endocrine pancreas: 35 years of research, but the enigma remains. *Endocrine Reviews* 28:84–116.

Gruetter R. 2003. Glycogen: the forgotten cerebral energy store. *J Neurosci Res* 74:179–183.

Gustavson SM, Chu SA, Nishizawa M, Farmer B, Neal D, Yang Y, Vaughan S, Donahue EP, Flakoll P, Cherrington AD. 2003. Glucagon's actions are modified by the combination of epinephrine and gluconeogenic precursor infusion. *Am J Physiol Endocrinol Metab* 285:E534–E544.

Gürlek A, Erbas T, Gedik O. 1999. Frequency of severe hypoglycaemia in type 1 and type 2 diabetes during conventional insulin therapy. *Exp Clin Endocrinol Diabetes* 107:220–224.

Haymond MW, Schreiner B. 2001. Mini-dose glucagon rescue to children with type 1 diabetes. *Diabetes Care* 24:643–645.

Heller SR, Cryer PE. 1991a. Hypoinsulinemia is not critical to glucose recovery from hypoglycemia in humans. *Am J Physiol Endocrinol Metab* 261:E41–E48.

———. 1991b. Reduced neuroendocrine and symptomatic responses to subsequent hypoglycemia after 1 episode of hypoglycemia in nondiabetic humans. *Diabetes* 40:223–226.

Henderson JN, Allen KV, Deary IJ, Frier BM. 2003. Hypoglycaemia in insulin-treated type 2 diabetes: frequency, symptoms and impaired awareness. *Diabet Med* 20:1016–1021.

Hepburn DA, MacLeod KM, Pell AC, Scougal IJ, Frier BM. 1993. Frequency and symptoms of hypoglycaemia experienced by patients with type 2 diabetes treated with insulin. *Diabet Med* 10:231–237.

Hershey T, Perantie DC, Warren SL, Zimmerman EC, Sadler M, White NH. 2005. Frequency and timing of severe hypoglycemia affects spatial memory in children with type 1 diabetes. *Diabetes Care* 28:2372–2377.

Herzog RI, Chan O, Yu S, Dziura J, McNay EC, Sherwin RS. 2008. Effect of acute and recurrent hypoglycemia on changes in brain glycogen concentration. *Endocrinology* 149:1499–1504.

Hirsch IB. 2005. Insulin analogues. *N Engl J Med* 352:174–183.

Hirsch IB, Marker JC, Smith L, Spina RJ, Parvin CA, Holloszy JO, Cryer PE. 1991. Insulin and glucagon in the prevention of hypoglycemia during exercise in humans. *Am J Physiol Endocrinol Metab* 260:E695–E704.

Hoffman RP, Singer-Granick C, Drash AL, Becker DJ. 1994. Abnormal alpha cell hypoglycemic recognition in children with insulin dependent diabetes mellitus (IDDM). *J Pediatr Endocrinol* 7:225–234.

Holman RR, Paul SK, Ethel MA, Matthews DR, Neil HAW. 2008. 10-year follow-up of intensive glucose control in type 2 diabetes. *N Engl J Med* 359:1577-1589.

Holstein A, Egberts EH. 2003. Risk of hypoglycaemia with oral antidiabetic agents in patients with type 2 diabetes. *Exp Clin Endocrinol Metab* 111:405–414.

Holstein A, Plaschke A, Böttcher Y, Stumvoll M, Kovacs P. 2006. The insertion/deletion polymorphism in the angiotensin-converting enzyme gene and hypoglycemia awareness in patients with type 1 diabetes. *Horm Metab Res* 38:603–606.

Holstein A, Plaschke A, Egberts E-H. 2003. Clinical characterization of severe hypoglycaemia: a prospective population-based study. *Exp Clin Endocrinol Diabetes* 111:364–369.

Horvath K, Jeitler K, Berghold A, Ebrahim SH, Gratzer TW, Plank J, Kaiser T, Pieber TR, Siebenhofer A. 2007. Long-acting insulin analogues versus NPH insulin (human isophane insulin) for type 2 diabetes. *Cochrane Database of Systematic Reviews*. Issue 2. Art. No. CD005613. DOI: 10.1002/14651858.CD005613.pub3.

Hovorka R. 2005. Continuous glucose monitoring and closed-loop systems. *Diabet Med* 23:1–12.

Hyder F, Patel AB, Gjedde A, Rothman DL, Behar KL, Shulman RG. 2006. Neuronal-glial glucose oxidation and glutaminergic-GABAergic function. *J Cerebr Blood Flow Metab* 26:865–877.

Ipp E, Dobbs RE, Arimura A, Vale W, Harris V, Unger RH. 1977. Release of immunoreactive somatostatin from the pancreas in response to glucose, amino acids, pancreozymin-cholecystokinin, and tolbutamide. *J Clin Invest* 60:760–765.

Israelian Z, Gosmanov NR, Szoke E, Schorr M, Bokhari S, Cryer PE, Gerich JE, Meyer C. 2005. Increasing the decrement in intraislet insulin improves glucagon responses to hypoglycemia in advanced type 2 diabetes. *Diabetes Care* 28:2691–2696.

Itoh Y, Esaki T, Shimoji K, Cook M, Law MJ, Kaufman E, Sokoloff L. 2003. Dichloroacetate effects on glucose and lactate oxidation by neurons and astroglia in vitro and on glucose utilization by brain in vivo. *Proc Natl Acad Sci U S A* 100:4879–4884.

Jacobsen AM. 1996. The psychological care of patients with insulin-dependent diabetes mellitus. *N Engl J Med* 344:1249–1253.

Jaferi A, Bhatnagar S. 2006. Corticosterone can act at the posterior paraventricular thalamus to inhibit hypothalamic-pituitary-adrenal activity in animals that habituate to repeated stress. *Endocrinology* 147:4917–4930.

Jeitler K, Horvath K, Berghold A, Gratzer TW, Neeser K, Pieber TR, Siebenhofer A. 2008. Continuous subcutaneous insulin infusion versus multiple daily injections in patients with diabetes mellitus: systematic review and meta-analysis. *Diabetologia* 51:941–951.

Jones TW, Porter P, Sherwin RS, Davis EA, O'Leary P, Frazer F, Byrne G, Stick S, Tamborlane WV. 1998. Decreased epinephrine responses to hypoglycemia during sleep. *N Engl J Med* 338:1657–1662.

Kahn KJ, Myers RE. 1971. Insulin induced hypoglycaemia in the non-human primate. I. Clinical consequences. In *Brain Hypoxia*. Brierley JB, Meldrum BS, Eds. London, William Heinemann Medical Books, pp. 185–194.

Kern W, Peters A, Fruehwald-Schultes B, Deininger E, Born J, Fehm HL. 2001. Improving influence of insulin on cognitive functions in humans. *Neuroendocrinology* 74:270–280.

Kilpatrick ES, Rigby AS, Goode K, Atkin SL. 2007. Relating mean blood glucose and glucose variability to the risk of multiple episodes of hypoglycaemia in type 1 diabetes. *Diabetologia* 50:2553–2561.

Knudsen GM, Hasselbach SG, Hertz MM, Paulson OB. 1999. High dose insulin does not increase glucose transfer across the blood-brain barrier in humans: a re-evaluation. *Eur J Clin Invest* 29:687–691.

Kovatchev BP, Cox DJ, Gonder-Frederick LA, Young-Hyman D, Schlundt D, Clarke WL. 1998. Assessment of risk for severe hypoglycemia among adults with IDDM: validation of the low blood glucose index. *Diabetes Care* 21:1870–1875.

Kovatchev BP, Cox DJ, Kumar A, Gonder-Frederick LA, Clarke WL. 2003. Algorithmic evaluation of metabolic control and risk of severe hypoglycemia in type 1 and type 2 diabetes using self-monitoring blood glucose (SMBG) data. *Diabetes Technol Ther* 5:817–828.

Lachin JM, Genuth S, Nathan DM, Zinman B, Rutledge BN, for the DCCT/EDIC Research Group. 2008. Effect of glycemic exposure on the risk of microvascular complications in the Diabetes Control and Complications Trial: revisited. *Diabetes* 57:995–1001.

Laing SP, Swerdlow AJ, Slater SD, Botha JL, Burden AC, Waugh NR, Smith AWM, Hill RD, Bingley PJ, Patterson CC, Qiao Z, Keen H. 1999. The British Diabetic Association Cohort Study. I. All-cause mortality in patients with insulin-treated diabetes mellitus. *Diabetic Med* 16:459–465.

Laitinen T, Lyyra-Laitinen T, Huopio H, Vauhkonen I, Halonen T, Hartikainen J, Niskanen L, Laakso M. 2008. Electrocardiographic alterations during hyperinsulinemic hypoglycemia in healthy subjects. *Ann Noninvasive Electrocardiol* 13:97–105.

Lee SP, Yeoh L, Harris ND, Davies CM, Robinson RT, Leathard A, Newman C, Macdonald IA, Heller SR. 2004. Influence of autonomic neuropathy on QTc interval lengthening during hypoglycemia in type 1 diabetes. *Diabetes* 53:1535–1542.

Leese GP, Wang J, Broomhall J, Kelly P, Marsden A, Morrison W, Frier BM, Morris AD, DARTS/MEMO Collaboration. 2003. Frequency of severe hypoglycemia requiring emergency treatment in type 1 and type 2 diabetes: a population based study of health service resource use. *Diabetes Care* 26:1176–1180.

Levin BE, Becker TC, Eiki J, Zhang BB, Dunn-Meynell AA. 2008. Ventromedial hypothalamic glucokinase is an important mediator of the counterregulatory response to insulin-induced hypoglycemia. *Diabetes* 57:1371–1379.

Lubow JM, Piñón IG, Avogaro A, Cobelli C, Treeson DM, Mandeville KA, Toffolo G, Boyle PJ. 2006. Brain oxygen utilization is unchanged by hypoglycemia in normal humans: lactate, alanine, and leucine uptake are not sufficient to offset energy deficit. *Am J Physiol Endocrinol Metab* 290:E149–E153.

Lüddeke H-J, Sreenan S, Aczel S, Maxeiner S, Yeniqun M, Kozlovski P, Gydesen H, Dornhorst A, on behalf of the PREDICTIVE Study Group. 2007. PREDICTIVE: A global, prospective observational study to evaluate insulin detemir treatment in types 1 and 2 diabetes: baseline characteristics and predictors of hypoglycemia from the European cohort. *Diabetes Obes Metab* 9:428–434.

MacCuish AC. 1993. Treatment of hypoglycemia. In *Diabetes and Hypoglycemia*. Frier BM, Fisher BM, Eds. London, Edward Arnold, pp. 212–221.

MacDonald MJ. 1987. Post exercise late onset hypoglycemia in insulin-dependent diabetic patients. *Diabetes Care* 10:584–588.

MacDonald PE, De Marinis YZ, Ramracheya R, Salehi A, Ma X, Johnson PRV, Cox R, Eliasson L, Rorsman P. 2007. A $K_{ATP}$ channel dependent pathway within α cells regulates glucagon release from both rodent and human islets of Langerhans. *PLoS Biology* 5:1236–1247.

MacGorman LR, Rizza RA, Gerich JE. 1981. Physiological concentrations of growth hormone exert insulin-like and insulin antagonistic effects on both hepatic and extra-hepatic tissues in man. *J Clin Endocrinol Metab* 53:556–559.

MacLeod KM, Hepburn DA, Frier BM. 1993. Frequency and morbidity of severe hypoglycaemia in insulin-treated diabetic patients. *Diabet Med* 10:238–245.

Maggs DG, Jacob R, Rife F, Caprio S, Tamborlane WV, Sherwin RS. 1997. Counterregulation in peripheral tissues. *Diabetes* 46:70–76.

Marker JC, Hirsch IB, Smith L, Parvin CA, Holloszy JO, Cryer PE. 1991. Catecholamines in the prevention of hypoglycemia during exercise in humans. *Am J Physiol Endocrinol Metab* 260:E705–E712.

Marty N, Dallaporta M, Thorens B. 2007. Brain glucose sensing, counterregulation and energy homeostasis. *Physiology* 22:241–251.

Maruyama H, Hisatomi A, Orci L, Grodsky GM, Unger RH. 1984. Insulin within islets is a physiologic glucagon release inhibitor. *J Clin Invest* 74:2296–2299.

Mason GF, Petersen KF, Lebon V, Rothman DL, Shulman GI. 2006. Increased brain monocarboxylic acid transport and utilization in type 1 diabetes. *Diabetes* 55:929–934.

McCrimmon R. 2008. The mechanisms that underlie glucose sensing during hypoglycaemia in diabetes. *Diabet Med* 25:513–522.

McCrimmon RJ, Deary IJ, Gold AE, Hepburn DA, MacLeod KM, Ewing FME, Frier BM. 2003a. Symptoms reported during experimental hypoglycaemia: effect of method of induction of hypoglycaemia and of diabetes *per se. Diabet Med* 20:507–509.

McCrimmon RJ, Evans ML, Fan X, McNay E, Chan O, Ding Y, Zhu W, Gram DX, Sherwin RS. 2005. Activation of ATP-sensitive K$^+$ channels in the ventromedial hypothalamus amplifies counterregulatory hormone responses to hypoglycemia in normal and recurrently hypoglycemic rats. *Diabetes* 54:3169–3174.

McCrimmon R, Jacob RJ, Fan X, McNay EC, Sherwin RS. 2003b. Effects of recurrent antecedent hypoglycaemia and chronic hyperglycaemia on brainstem extra-cellular glucose concentrations during acute hypoglycaemia in conscious diabetic BB rats. *Diabetologia* 46:1658–1661.

McCrimmon RJ, Shaw M, Fan X, Cheng H, Ding Y, Vella M, Zhou L, McNay E, Sherwin RS. 2008. Key role for AMP-activated protein kinase in the ventromedial hypothalamus in regulating counterregulatory hormone responses to acute hypoglycemia. *Diabetes* 57:444–450.

McCrimmon RJ, Song Z, Cheng H, McNay EC, Weikart-Yeckel C, Fan X, Routh VH, Sherwin RS. 2006. Corticotrophin-releasing factor receptors within the ventromedial hypothalamus regulate hypoglycemia-induced hormonal counterregulation. *J Clin Invest* 116:1723–1730.

McGregor VP, Banarer S, Cryer PE. 2002. Elevated endogenous cortisol reduces autonomic neuroendocrine and symptom responses to subsequent hypoglycemia. *Am J Physiol Endocrinol Metab* 282:E770-E777.

McNay EC, Sherwin RS. 2004. Effect of recurrent hypoglycemia on spatial cognition and cognitive metabolism in normal and diabetic rats. *Diabetes* 53:418–425.

Meyer C, Grossman R, Mitrakou A, Mahler R, Veneman T, Gerich J, Bretzel RG. 1998. Effects of autonomic neuropathy on counterregulation and awareness of hypoglycemia in type 1 diabetic patients. *Diabetes Care* 21:1920–1966.

Mitrakou A, Ryan C, Veneman T, Mokan M, Jenssen T, Kiss I, Durrant J, Cryer P, Gerich J. 1991. Hierarchy of glycemic thresholds for counterregulatory hormone secretion, symptoms and cerebral dysfunction. *Am J Physiol Endocrinol Metab* 260:E67–E74.

Mühlhauser I, Overmann H, Bender R, Bott U, Berger M. 1997. Risk factors for severe hypoglycaemia in adult patients with type 1 diabetes: a prospective population based study. *Diabetologia* 41:1274–1282.

Mukhopadhyay A, Farrell T, Fraser RB, Ola B. 2007. Continuous subcutaneous insulin infusion vs intensive conventional insulin therapy in pregnant diabetic women: a systematic review and metaanalysis of randomized, controlled trials. *Am J Obstet Gynecol* 197:447–456.

Mundinger TO, Mei Q, Figlewicz DP, Lernmark A, Taborsky GJ Jr. 2003. Impaired glucagon response to sympathetic nerve stimulation in the BB diabetic rat: effect of early sympathetic islet neuropathy. *Am J Physiol Endocrinol Metab* 285:E1047–E1054.

Murata GH, Duckworth WC, Shah JH, Wendel CS, Mohler MJ, Hoffman RM. 2005. Hypoglycemia in stable, insulin-treated veterans with type 2 diabetes: a prospective study of 1662 episodes. *J Diabetes Complications* 19:10–17.

Nielsen LR, Pedersen-Bjergaard U, Thorsteinsson B, Johansen M, Damm P, Mathiesen ER. 2008. Hypoglycemia in pregnant women with type 1 diabetes. *Diabetes Care* 31:9–14.

Nordfeldt S, Ludvigsson J. 2005. Fear and other disturbances of severe hypoglycaemia in children and adolescents with type 1 diabetes mellitus. *J Pediatr Endocrinol Metab* 18:83–91.

Nordfeldt S, Samuelsson U. 2003. Serum ACE predicts severe hypoglycemia in children and adolescents with type 1 diabetes. *Diabetes Care* 26:274–278.

Obici S, Zhang BB, Karkanias G, Rossetti L. 2002. Hypothalamic insulin signaling is required for inhibition of glucose production. *Nat Med* 8:1376–1382.

Ohkubo Y, Kishikawa H, Araki E, Miyata T, Isami S, Motoyoshi S, Kojima Y, Furuyoshi N, Shichiri M. 1995. Intensive insulin therapy prevents the progression of diabetic microvascular complications in Japanese patients with non-insulin dependent diabetes mellitus: a randomized prospective 6-year study. *Diabetes Res Clin Pract* 28:103–117.

Olsen HL, Theander S, Bokvist K, Buschard K, Wollheim CB, Gromada J. 2005. Glucose stimulates glucose release in single rat α-cells by mechanisms that mirror the stimulus-secretion coupling in β-cells. *Endocrinology* 146:4861–4870.

Ovalle F, Fanelli CG, Paramore DS, Hershey T, Craft S, Cryer PE. 1998. Brief twice-weekly episodes of hypoglycemia reduce detection of clinical hypoglycemia in type 1 diabetes mellitus. *Diabetes* 47:1472–1479.

Owen OE, Felig P, Morgan AP, Wahren J, Cahill GF. 1969. Liver and kidney metabolism during prolonged starvation. *J Clin Invest* 48:574–583.

Öz G, Seaquist ER, Kumar A, Criego AB, Benedict LE, Rao JP, Henry P-G, Van De Moortele P-F, Gruetter R. 2007. Human brain glycogen content and metabolism: implications on its role in brain energy metabolism. *Am J Physiol Endocrinol Metab* 292:E946–E951.

Paramore DS, Fanelli CG, Shah SD, Cryer PE. 1998. Forearm norepinephrine spillover during standing, hyperinsulinemia and hypoglycemia. *Am J Physiol Endocrinol Metab* 275:E872–E881.

Pedersen-Bjergaard U, Agerholm-Larsen B, Pramming S, Hougaard P, Thorsteinsson B. 2001. Activity of angiotensin-converting enzyme and risk of severe hypoglycemia in type 1 diabetes mellitus. *Lancet* 357:1248–1253.

———. 2003. Prediction of severe hypoglycaemia by angiotensin-converting enzyme activity and genotype in type 1 diabetes. *Diabetologia* 46:89–96.

Pedersen-Bjergaard U, Høi-Hansen T, Thorsteinsson B. 2007. An evaluation of methods of assessing impaired awareness of hypoglycemia in type 1 diabetes. *Diabetes Care* 30:e112.

Pedersen-Bjergaard U, Pramming S, Thorsteinsson B. 2003. Recall of severe hypoglycemia and self-estimated state of awareness in type 1 diabetes. *Diabetes Metab Res Rev* 19:232–240.

Perantie DC, Wu J, Koller JM, Lim A, Warren SL, Black KJ, Sadler M, White NH, Hershey T. 2007. Regional brain volume differences associated with hyperglycemia and severe hypoglycemia in youth with type 1 diabetes. *Diabetes Care* 30:2331–2337.

Polonsky KS, Licinio-Paixao J, Given BD, Pugh W, Rue P, Galloway J, Karrison T, Frank B. 1986. Use of biosynthetic human C-peptide in the measurement of insulin secretion rates in normal volunteers and type I diabetic patients. *J Clin Invest* 77:98–105.

Porte D Jr, Baskin DG, Schwartz MW. 2005. Insulin signaling in the central nervous system: a critical role in metabolic homeostasis and disease from *C. elegans* to humans. *Diabetes* 54:1264–1276.

Pramming S, Thorsteinsson B, Bendtson I, Binder C. 1991. Symptomatic hypoglycaemia in 411 type 1 diabetic patients. *Diabet Med* 8:217–222.

Preiser J-C, Devos P. 2007. Clinical experience with tight glucose control by intensive insulin therapy. *Crit Care Med* 35 (Suppl.):S503–S507.

Qaseem A, Vijan S, Snow V, Cross JT, Weiss KB, Owens DK, for the Clinical Efficacy Assessment Subcommittee of the American College of Physicians. 2007. Glycemic control and type 2 diabetes mellitus: the optimal hemoglobin $A_{1C}$

targets: a guidance statement from the American College of Physicians. *Ann Intern Med* 147:417–422.

Raju B, Arbelaez AM, Breckenridge SM, Cryer PE. 2006. Nocturnal hypoglycemia in type 1 diabetes: an assessment of preventive bedtime treatments. *J Clin Endocrinol Metab* 91:2087-2092.

Raju B, Cryer PE. 2005. Loss of the decrement in intraislet insulin plausibly explains loss of the glucagon response to hypoglycemia in insulin-deficient diabetes. *Diabetes* 54:757–764.

Raju B, McGregor VP, Cryer PE. 2003. Cortisol elevations comparable to those that occur during hypoglycemia do not cause hypoglycemia-associated autonomic failure. *Diabetes* 52:2083–2089.

Reichard P, Pihl M. 1994. Mortality and treatment side-effects during long-term intensified conventional insulin treatment in the Stockholm Diabetes Intervention Study. *Diabetes* 43:313–317.

Rickels MR, Schutta MH, Mueller R, Kapoor S, Markmann JF, Naji A, Teff KL. 2007. Glycemic thresholds for activation of counterregulatory hormone and symptom responses in islet transplant recipients. *J Clin Endocrinol Metab* 92:873–879.

Rizza RA, Cryer PE, Gerich JE. 1979. Role of glucagon, catecholamines, and growth hormone in human glucose counterregulation. *J Clin Invest* 64:62–71.

Rizza RA, Cryer PE, Haymond MW, Gerich JE. 1980. Adrenergic mechanisms for the effect of epinephrine on glucose production and clearance in man. *J Clin Invest* 65:682–689.

Rizza RA, Mandarino L, Gerich J. 1982. Cortisol-induced insulin resistance in man: impaired suppression of glucose production and stimulation of glucose utilization due to a post-receptor defect of insulin action. *J Clin Endocrinol Metab* 54:131–138.

Rosen SG, Clutter WE, Berk MA, Shah SD, Cryer PE. 1984. Epinephrine supports the postabsorptive plasma glucose concentration and prevents hypoglycemia when glucagon secretion is deficient in man. *J Clin Invest* 73:405–411.

Rossetti P, Porcellati F, Bolli GB, Fanelli CG. 2008. Prevention of hypoglycemia while achieving good glycemic control in type 1 diabetes. *Diabetes Care* 31 (Suppl. 2):S113–S120.

Samols E, Stagner JI, Ewart RBL, Marks V. 1988. The order of islet microvascular cellular perfusion is B→A→D in the perfused rat pancreas. *J Clin Invest* 82:350–353.

Samols E, Tyler J, Marks V. 1972. Glucagon-insulin interrelationships. In *Glucagon: Molecular Physiology, Clinical and Therapeutic Implications.* Lefebvre P, Unger RH, Eds. Elmsford, N.Y., Pergamon Press, pp. 151–174.

Sanders NM, Wilkinson CW, Taborsky GJ Jr, Al-Noori S, Daumen W, Zavosh A, Figlewicz DP. 2008. The selective serotonin reuptake inhibitor sertraline enhances counterregulatory responses to hypoglycemia. *Am J Physiol Endocrinol Metab* 294:E853–E860.

Sandoval DA, Aftab Guy DL, Richardson MA, Ertl AC, Davis SN. 2004. Effects of low and moderate antecedent exercise on counterregulatory responses to subsequent hypoglycemia in type 1 diabetes. *Diabetes* 53:1798–1806.

Saudek CD, Duckworth WC, Giobbie-Hurder A, Henderson WG, Henry RR, Kelley DE, Edelman SV, Zieve FJ, Adler RA, Anderson JW, Anderson RJ, Hamilton BP, Donner TW, Kirkman MS, Morgan NA. 1996. Implantable insulin pump vs. multiple dose insulin for non-insulin dependent diabetes mellitus: a randomized clinical trial. *J Am Med Assoc* 276:1322–1327.

Schultes B, Jauch-Chara K, Gais S, Hallschmid M, Reiprich E, Kern W, Oltmanns KM, Peters A, Fehm HL, Born J. 2007. Defective awakening response to nocturnal hypoglycemia in patients with type 1 diabetes mellitus. *PLoS Medicine* 4:e69.

Schultes B, Oltmanns KM, Kern W, Fehm HL, Born J, Peters A. 2003. Modulation of hunger by plasma glucose and metformin. *J Clin Endocrinol Metab* 88:1133–1141.

Schwartz NS, Clutter WE, Shah SD, Cryer PE. 1987. Glycemic thresholds for activation of glucose counterregulatory systems are higher than the threshold for symptoms. *J Clin Invest* 79:777–781.

Seaquist ER, Damberg GS, Tkac I, Gruetter R. 2001. The effect of insulin on in vivo cerebral glucose concentrations and rates of glucose transport/metabolism in humans. *Diabetes* 50:2203–2209.

Segel SA, Fanelli CG, Dence CS, Markham J, Videen TO, Paramore DS, Powers WJ, Cryer PE. 2001. Blood-to-brain glucose transport, cerebral glucose metabolism and cerebral blood flow are not increased following hypoglycemia. *Diabetes* 50:1911–1917.

Segel SA, Paramore DS, Cryer PE. 2002. Hypoglycemia-associated autonomic failure in advanced type 2 diabetes. *Diabetes* 51:724–733.

Service FJ, Rizza RA, Zimmerman BR, Dyck PJ, O'Brien PC, Melton LJ III. 1997. The classification of diabetes by clinical and C-peptide criteria. *Diabetes Care* 20:198–201.

Sherck SM, Shiota M, Saccomando J, Cardin S, Allen EJ, Hastings JR, Neal DW, Williams PE, Cherrington AD. 2001. Pancreatic response to mild non-insulin induced hypoglycemia does not involve extrinsic neural input. *Diabetes* 50:2487–2496.

Sherwin RS. 2008. Bringing light to the dark side of diabetes. A journey across the blood-brain barrier. *Diabetes* 57:2259–2267.

Skrivarhaug T, Bangstad H-J, Stene LC, Sandvik L, Hanssen KF, Joner G. 2006. Long-term mortality in a nationwide cohort of childhood-onset type 1 diabetic patients in Norway. *Diabetologia* 49:298–305.

Steffes MW, Sibley S, Jackson M, Thomas W. 2003. β-Cell function and the development of diabetes related complications in the Diabetes Control and Complications Trial. *Diabetes Care* 26:832–836.

Steil GM, Rebrin K, Darwin C, Hariri F, Saad MF. 2006. Feasibility of automating insulin delivery for the treatment of type 1 diabetes. *Diabetes* 55:3344–3350.

Stettler C, Allemann S, Jüni P, Cull CA, Holman RR, Egger M, Krähenbühl S, Diem P. 2006. Glycemic control and macrovascular disease in types 1 and 2 diabetes: meta-analysis of randomized trials. *Am Heart J* 152:27–38.

Suh SW, Gum ET, Hamby AM, Chan PH, Swanson RA. 2007. Hypoglycemic neuronal death is triggered by glucose reperfusion and activation of neuronal NADPH oxidase. *J Clin Invest* 117:910–918.

Taborsky GJ Jr, Ahrén B, Havel PJ. 1998. Autonomic mediation of glucagon secretion during hypoglycemia. *Diabetes* 47:995–1005.

Tansey MJ, Tsalikian E, Beck RW, Mauras N, Buckingham BA, Weinzimer SA, Janz KF, Kollman C, Xing D, Ruedy KJ, Steffes MW, Borland TM, Singh RJ, Tamborlane WV, for the Diabetes Research in Children Network (DirecNet) Study Group. 2006. The effects of aerobic exercise on glucose and counterregulatory hormone concentrations in children with type 1 diabetes. *Diabetes Care* 29:20–25.

Teves D, Videen TO, Cryer PE, Powers WJ. 2004. Activation of human medial prefrontal cortex during autonomic responses to hypoglycemia. *Proc Natl Acad Sci U S A* 101:6217–6221.

Towler DA, Havlin CE, Craft S, Cryer PE. 1993. Mechanism of awareness of hypoglycemia: perception of neurogenic (predominantly cholinergic) rather than neuroglycopenic symptoms. *Diabetes* 42:1791–1798.

Tsalikian E, Mauras N, Beck RW, Tamborlane WV, Janz KF, Chase HP, Wysocki T, Weinzimer SA, Buckingham BA,

Kollman C, Xing D, Ruedy KJ, for the Diabetes Research in Network (DirecNet) Study Group. 2005. Impact of exercise on overnight glycemic control in children with type 1 diabetes. *J Pediatr* 147:528–534.

Tse TF, Clutter WE, Shah SD, Cryer PE. 1983b. Mechanisms of postprandial glucose counterregulation in man: physiologic roles of glucagon and epinephrine vis-à-vis insulin in the prevention of hypoglycemia late after glucose ingestion. *J Clin Invest* 72:278–286.

Tse TF, Clutter WE, Shah SD, Miller JP, Cryer PE. 1983a. Neuroendocrine responses to glucose ingestion in man: specificity, temporal relationships and quantitative aspects. *J Clin Invest* 72:270–277.

Tunbridge WMG. 1981. Factors contributing to deaths of diabetics under 50 years of age. *Lancet* 2:569–572.

U.K. Hypoglycaemia Study Group [UK Hypo Group]. 2007. Risk of hypoglycaemia in types 1 and 2 diabetes: effects of treatment modalities and their duration. *Diabetologia* 50:1140–1147.

U.K. Prospective Diabetes Study Group [UKPDS]. 1995. Overview of 6 years of therapy of type II diabetes: a progressive disease. *Diabetes* 44:1249–1258.

———. 1998a. Intensive blood-glucose control with sulphonylureas or insulin compared with conventional treatment and risk of complications in patients with type 2 diabetes (UKPDS 33). *Lancet* 352:837–853.

————. 1998b. Effect of intensive blood-glucose control with metformin on complications in overweight patients with type 2 diabetes (UKPDS 34). *Lancet* 352:854–865.

————. 1998c. United Kingdom Prospective Diabetes Study 24: a six year, randomized, controlled trial comparing sulfonylurea, insulin and metformin therapy in patients with newly diagnosed type 2 diabetes that could not be controlled with diet therapy. *Ann Intern Med* 128:165–175.

Vallbo AB, Hagbarth K-E, Wallin BG. 2004. Microneurography: how the technique developed and its role in the investigation of the sympathetic nervous system. *J Appl Physiol* 96:1262–1269.

Van den Berghe G, Wilmer A, Hermans G, Meersseman W, Wouters PJ, Milants I, Van Wijngaerden E, Bobbaers H, Bouillon R. 2006. Intensive insulin therapy in the medical ICU. *N Engl J Med* 354:449–461.

Van den Berghe G, Wouters P, Weekers F, Verwaest C, Bruyninckx F, Schetz M, Vlasselaers D, Ferdinande P, Lauwers P, Bouillon R. 2001. Intensive insulin therapy in critically ill patients. *N Engl J Med* 345:1359–1367.

Wahren J, Ekberg K, Fernqvist-Forbes E, Nair S. 1999. Brain substrate utilization during acute hypoglycaemia. *Diabetologia* 42:812–818.

Whipple AO. 1938. The surgical therapy of hyperinsulinism. *J Int Chir* 3:237–276.

White NH, Skor DA, Cryer PE, Levandoski LA, Bier DM, Santiago JV. 1983. Identification of type 1 diabetic patients at increased risk for hypoglycemia during intensive therapy. *N Engl J Med* 308:485–491.

Wiethop BV, Cryer PE. 1993a. Glycemic actions of alanine and terbutaline in IDDM. *Diabetes Care* 16:1124–1130.

———. 1993b. Alanine and terbutaline in the treatment of hypoglycemia in IDDM. *Diabetes Care* 16:1131–1136.

Wild S, Roglic G, Green A, Sicree R, King H. 2004. Global prevalence of diabetes: estimates for the year 2000 and projections for 2030. *Diabetes Care* 27:1047–1053.

Wilson DM, Beck RW, Tamborlane WV, Dontchev MJ, Kollman C, Chase P, Fox LA, Ruedy KJ, Tsalikian E, Weinzimer SA, The DirecNet Study Group. 2007. The accuracy of the FreeStyle Navigator continuous glucose monitoring system in children with type 1 diabetes. *Diabetes Care* 30:59–64.

Wright AD, Cull CA, MacLeod KM, Holman RR, for the UKPDS Group. 2006. Hypoglycemia in type 2 diabetic patients randomized to and maintained on monotherapy with diet, sulfonylurea, metformin, or insulin for 6 years from diagnosis: UKPDS73. *J Diabetes Complications* 20:395–401.

Wurtman RJ. 2002. Stress and the adrenocortical control of epinephrine synthesis. *Metabolism* 51:11–14.

Wurtman RJ, Axelrod J. 1965. Adrenaline synthesis: control by the pituitary gland and adrenal glucocorticoids. *Science* 150:1464–1465.

Yki-Järvinen H, Ryysy L, Nikkilä K, Tulokas T, Vanamo R, Heikkilä M. 1999. Comparison of bedtime insulin regimens in patients with type 2 diabetes mellitus. *Ann Intern Med* 130:389–396.

Zammitt N, Geddes J, Warren RE, Marioni R, Ashby PJ, Frier BM. 2007. Serum angiotensin-converting enzyme and frequency of severe hypoglycaemia in type 1 diabetes: does a relationship exist? *Diabet Med* 24:1449–1454.

Zhou L, Fan X, Ding Y, Zhu W, Chan O, Vella MC, Sherwin RS, McCrimmon RJ. 2007. Acute hypoglycemia induces activated neurons in the lateral hypothalamus of the brain and the intermediolateral cell column of the spinal cord, while recurrent hypoglycemia blunts them (Abstract). *Diabetes* 56:A101.

Zhou H, Tran PO, Yang S, Zhang T, Le Roy E, Oseid E, Robertson RP. 2004. Regulation of alpha-cell function by the beta-cell during hypoglycemia in Wistar rats: the "switch-off" hypothesis. *Diabetes* 53:1482–1487.

Zhou H, Zhang T, Harmon JS, Bryan J, Robertson RP. 2007. Zinc, not insulin, regulates the rat alpha cell to hypoglycemia in vivo. *Diabetes* 56:1107–1112.

# Index

Note: Page numbers followed by *t* refer to tables. Page numbers followed by *f* refer to figures.

## A

α-glucosidase inhibitors, 3, 46, 105
A1C, 1–2, 13–14, 78*t*, 81, 95–97, 101*t*, 103
Acetylcholine (ACh), 23, 26–27, 29, 41*f,* 53
Action to Control Cardiovascular Risk in Diabetes
    [ACCORD] trial, 11, 13–14
Adrenal cortices, 29
Adrenal medullae, 22–23, 29–31, 61
Adrenergic
    activation, 26–27, 33
        agonist, 53
        terbutaline, 96
    blockade, 38–39, 63
    cutaneous vasoconstriction, 24
    receptors, 30, 33
    sensitivity, 53
    symptoms, 23
Adrenocortical cortisol deficiency, 29
Adrenomedullary, 23, 27, 40–41, 48, 52, 54, 63, 69. *See also*
    chromaffin cells; epinephrine

# C

types, 95–96

waning of, 35

Insulin dependent diabetes mellitus (IDDM). *See* diabetes, type 1 (T1DM)

Intra-islet hyperinsulinemia, 67

Intra-islet insulin hypothesis, 64*f,* 65–67

Islet δ-cells, 66

Islet microcirculation, 65

Islet transplantation, 61

Isoproterenol, 53

Isotope dilution, 31

# K

Ketoacidosis, 103

Ketones, 17

Kidneys, 21*t,* 24–25, 27, 32

# L

Lactate, 17–19, 32, 70

Lateral orbitofrontal cortex, 72

LDL cholesterol, 104

Leucine, 18

Lipolysis, 27

Liver, 18, 21*t,* 24*t,* 25–28, 32, 87

# M

Macrovascular, benefits of long-term glycemic control, 1, 9, 101

# S

# W

Weight loss, 78*t*, 79, 105
Whipple's triad, 2, 21, viii

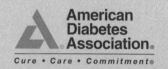

American
Diabetes
Association.
*Cure • Care • Commitment®*

# ADA's Medical Management Series:

Helping you focus on the most important patient symptoms and
assisting you in making the most accurate diagnosis

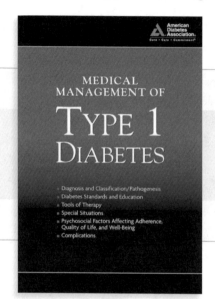

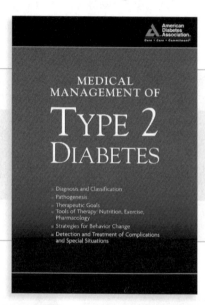

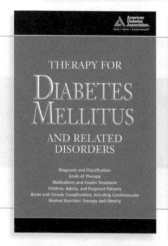

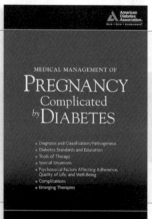

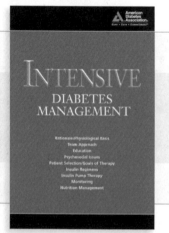

WITHDRAWN